HEALING TEAS

HOW TO PREPARE AND USE TEAS TO MAXIMIZE YOUR HEALTH

MARIE NADINE ANTOL

Avery Publishing Group
Garden City Park, New York

The procedures in this book are based upon the research and personal experiences of the author. If you have any questions regarding the appropriateness of any procedure or material mentioned, the author and publisher strongly suggest consulting a professional health-care advisor.

Because any material or procedure can be misused, the author and publisher are not responsible for any adverse effects or consequences resulting from the use of any of the preparations, materials, or procedures suggested in this book. However, the publisher believes that this information should be available to the public.

Cover Designers: William Gonzalez and Rudy Shur
Front Cover Photo: SuperStock, Inc.
Back Cover Photo: Courtesy of Charleston Tea Plantation, Wadmalaw
   Island, South Carolina, the only tea plantation in America
Typesetter: Bonnie Freid
Artist: Vicki Rae Chelf
Printer: Paragon Press, Honesdale, PA

Library of Congress Cataloging-in-Publication Data

Antol, Marie Nadine.
   Healing teas : how to prepare and use teas to maximize your health
/ by Marie Nadine Antol.
      p.   cm.
   Includes index.
   ISBN 0-89529-707-8
   1. Herbal teas—Therapeutic use.   I. Title.
   RM666.H33A57   1996
   615'.323166—dc20   95-20039
                                                         CIP

Copyright © 1996 by Marie Nadine Antol

Printed in the United States of America

10   9   8   7

Contents

Acknowledgments,   v

Preface,   vii

Introduction,   1

Part I   Using Teas

1. Traditional Sipping Teas,   9
2. Traditional Healing Teas,   27
3. Healing Teas Today,   47
4. Shopping for Healing Teas,   67
5. The ABCs of Herb Cultivation,   79

Part II   Selecting Teas

6. A Selection of Natural Medicinals for Brewing
   Healing Teas,   91
7. Conclusion,   219

Sources of Supplies,   225
Sources of Information,   227
Bibliography,   229
Index,   235

Acknowledgments

I am deeply indebted to the following people for sharing their expertise on various healing tea protocols:

First and foremost, I am most particularly grateful to Morgana, proprietress and guiding light of The Raven of Venice, California. She was my primary consultant on the American and European brewing herbs that comprise most of the healing teas in this book. Her vast knowlege of herbology, coupled with her long experience in dispensing the very finest of brewing herbs through her shop, made her counsel invaluable. Morgana not only read the manuscript with her expert eye, she provided some very real insight on a number of teas that I might have missed. This book is much, much richer than it would have been had she not been kind enough to give me so much time.

Thanks also go to the staff members at the Ayurvedic Health Center of Pacific Palisades, California, for supplying me with so much information on East Indian teas and the traditional healing herbs of India, and for a guided tour of their impressive facility.

My experienced consultant on the centuries-old whole-body tonic teas of China was James Rea-Bailey, who dispenses knowledge and Chinese healing teas at the Tea Garden Herbal Emporium of Venice and West Hollywood, California. His willingness to take time to discuss these sustaining and health-promoting teas with me is very much appreciated.

I appreciate, too, the efforts of David Porrello at Avery Publishing, who labored to make the measurements in this book consistent and accurate.

Preface

My love affair with tea began a very long time ago. I not only enjoy teas of all kinds, I appreciate their gentle effects. The earliest "treatment" my mother applied when one of us felt ill was a "nice cup of tea." She believed there was nothing a good brew couldn't fix. Considering everything I've discovered in the past twenty years, it seems as if mother was right.

Almost twenty-five years ago, I became personally interested in the healing power of teas. At that time, my niece experienced a dramatic turnaround in her health through diet and herb teas. Nutrition's role in health was not being discussed much back in the early '70s. I began to wonder what else medical science might have missed. Thus began my lifelong investigation of natural medicinals.

I have often wished for a book that included good basic information on healing teas. I've done a lot of research and have yet to find a single source that told me everything I needed to know. It's taken me a long time to piece everything together. In one way or another, in a purely personal "family" way, I've been "working" on this material for over twenty years now.

My immediate family has benefited countless times from a combination of healing teas and modern medicine. All four of my adult children still call home for advice on natural medicinals whenever something goes wrong. I'm a grandmother now. My small Number One (and only) grandson has already benefited from sips of some of gramma's healing brews. I hope you'll also benefit from what you'll learn in this book.

To those of you seeking solid information on the healing teas, this book is the answer. Part I encompasses a history of teas, including traditional teas, herbal teas, and healing teas, plus a whole lot more. In Chapter 1, Traditional Sipping Teas, you'll learn about the first cup of tea—brewed 5,000 years ago by an Emperor of China—as well as the ancient and quite beautiful Japanese tea ceremony, and the extravagant high teas of British royalty.

Although it's difficult to describe an appeal that's purely personal and necessarily subjective, I'll try to tell you what various teas taste like. From the traditional teas—like Earl Gray and English (or Irish) Breakfast—to the light and delicious herbal blends, I'll give you an inkling of what to expect with your first sip. If you're already a tea drinker, maybe you haven't yet sampled all the varieties available. If you think you don't like tea, I'm betting that you just haven't hit on the right blend yet. Either way, this chapter may encourage you to try something new in the sipping teas.

In Chapter 2, Traditional Healing Teas, I'll give you a look at the long history of healing teas, so ancient that their use predates recorded history, and show you how these time-tested medicinals can serve a useful place in your life. I'll walk you through old China and the Ayurvedic healing system of India. You'll look through a window into the past and see how the Greeks, Romans, and Middle Eastern peoples traditionally used healing teas. Then we'll trek on into medieval Europe and the British Isles before booking passage across the sea to Colonial America, which includes a glimpse into how the native American medicinals and old European remedies intermingled. Expect a side excursion down to South America. I'll even give you a look at the macrobiotic teas that have come to us from Japan.

In Chapter 3, Healing Teas Today, you'll see how ancient and modern come together. Here's where you'll learn of the instances where science has validated the old beliefs. You probably already know that the science of compounding natural medicinals predates orthodox medicine by millennia. There are many, many pharmaceutical drugs in use today that originated in a steaming cup of healing tea. I'll tell you how the progression of events has brought us to the stage where we are today.

You may be surprised to learn that today, alternative medical systems like herbology, homeopathy, chiropractic, apitherapy, and the time-tested Chinese and Ayurvedic methods of healing are slowly but surely being welcomed as complementary treatments that support allopathic (orthodox) medicine. It's no longer an either/or approach to healing.

For example, in Hong Kong, the locals routinely visit health centers where allopathic and alternative practitioners work side by side. In mainland China, where the old ways long prevailed, Western medicine isn't the stepchild any longer. In this broad-based approach to health care, the watchword is "whatever works." Such treatment centers are springing up in many areas of the United States. If your area does not have a facility in which Eastern and Western medicine are friends, you can still take advantage of a bit of the ancient wisdom simply by using some of the healing teas you'll learn about in this book.

You will also find various methods of preparing healing teas at home, including making infusions and decoctions, but we won't stop there. I'll also give you some of the old "receipts" for making everything from poultices to salves to sitz baths.

In Chapter 4, Shopping for Healing Teas, I'll introduce and explain the terms that are used to describe the properties of various herbs. Once you know the jargon, you'll easily be able to match an herb with its action when you're standing in a store looking at boxes upon boxes of various dried herb parts.

You'll also find some general guidelines for buying everything from tea bags targeted for specific ailments, to the herbal blends designed to taste good while they soothe and relax, to the dried herb parts you'll need to blend and brew your own remedies. I'll tell you what to look for—and what to watch out for—when making your selections. I'll introduce you to some preblended medicinal teas that have been prepared according to the ancient formulas, as well as some up-to-the-minute blends. I'll also tell you the many advantages of using the whole herbs instead of extracted components.

And, just in case you're really interested in making teas from scratch, Chapter 5, The ABCs of Herb Cultivation, will show you how to start a garden that will produce a bumper crop of the "fixings" for your own healing teas. This chapter provides a general overview on everything from growing your own herbs to harvesting, drying, preparing, and storing nature's bounty.

Part II is the heart of the book. Chapter 6, A Selection of Natural Medicinals for Brewing Healing Teas, includes an A to Z Trouble-Shooting Guide to help you identify the teas to use for specific conditions. Here you'll also learn about the natural pharmaceuticals you need to prepare selected healing teas, including one made from propolis, an ancient remedy brewed from a substance taken from the beehive. You'll learn what natural medicinal to use for what condition, what parts of the substance are used, the various ways of preparing a suitable home treatment with the specific medicinal, and how to employ the preparation for best results. If there are any cautions to be observed, I'll warn you in the material covering each individual medicinal.

By the time you have reached Chapter 7, Conclusion, you will have all of the herbal basics under your belt. Now it will be up to you to discriminate the best times to use your knowledge of teas. Whether you choose a relaxing brew to lull you to sleep, or a powerful decoction to speed recovery, you will now know how to put the gentle power of healing teas to use for you and your family.

Introduction

The wonderful world of tea is about to be opened unto you. If you already enjoy tea, I think you'll be fascinated by some little-known facts about your favorite beverage. If you have not yet been initiated into the pleasures of tea, perhaps this book will inspire you to take a taste. There is a simple beauty in the taking of tea. Somehow, relaxing with a cup of tea carries you away into the serenity of a bygone age. But there is more than beauty to taking tea; it can also be an act of healing.

I believe in supporting the body with nutritive and natural-healing substances. Nowhere is it written that the ancient time-tested medicinals and therapies and today's allopathic protocols cannot benefit one another. I not only believe they can, but that they should. To dismiss healing systems that have survived for thousands of years doesn't make sense. These ancient protocols have lasted for just one reason. They work.

I personally became interested in the quite extraordinary power the body has to heal itself—especially when it is adequately supported—almost a quarter of a century ago. Here's how it happened.

In 1972, my sister—the harried mother of six daughters all under fifteen years of age—sent her eldest daughter, Shelley, to me. I was working at home, had the time and inclination, and my sister was overburdened caring for her large family, which included a handicapped child and a baby. She was afraid she wouldn't be able to give Shelley the amount of attention she needed.

Shelley had been suffering from an unexplained and quite frightening loss of weight. In spite of wanting to eat, she had no appetite and *couldn't* eat. Her personality changed. Normally, "mother's helper," she fought and squabbled with her sisters. She was morose and had severe mood swings. Most frightening of all, she was wobbly on her feet and was constantly blinking and rubbing her eyes because her vision blurred.

Here's where medical science stepped in. Although Shelley had all the classic symptoms, it took a six-hour glucose tolerance test to confirm a diagnosis of hypoglycemia, or low blood sugar. Hypoglycemia is caused by excess insulin circulating through the bloodstream. The condition can be caused by eating too little, or eating the wrong things, thereby triggering the pancreas to produce too much insulin. It can also occur when a diabetic takes (or is given) too much insulin.

Shelley arrived at my home with a book—*Low Blood Sugar and You*—a definitive text on correcting hypoglycemia and bringing blood sugar into balance by purely dietary means. This is when I learned first-hand how spectacularly the body can heal itself when properly supported by natural means.

I served Shelley high-protein mini-meals with an ounce or two of herb tea to wash them down. In the beginning, she needed coaxing because it was hard for her to eat. But, as her body began functioning better, she regained her appetite little-by-little. I was cooking three meals a day for my husband and four children, but I ate exactly the same foods I was serving Shelley. This grand body-normalizing program caused me to lose about ten pounds (happy day), while Shelley gradually gained back the almost twenty pounds she had lost. When I returned Shelley to her family, she was fully recovered and able to eat whatever she wished, within reason.

The turnaround Shelley experienced was stunning. And it was all accomplished by the simplest and most natural means imaginable. Back then (1974), medical science wasn't saying much of anything about the nutritional needs of the body. I began to wonder what else medical professionals were missing.

That was the beginning of my lifelong investigation of the natural healing substances employed by the ancients. Since that time, I have travelled throughout Europe and to the East, visiting, talking, sampling, experimenting, judging, and using teas that heal and other natural medicinals to support myself and my family through various illnesses.

My niece Shelley eventually became a convert to the natural ways, but she took a lot of convincing. She grew into a bright, beautiful—and stubborn—young woman. When she was pregnant with her first child, she began suffering from horrific migraine headaches. Because she didn't want to take anything that could potentially harm the child she was carrying, Shelley decided to tough it out. I recommended feverfew tea, but she scoffed at the notion that a simple little herb could be of help. I warned her that the effects of feverfew are cumulative and urged her to start taking the tea immediately as a preventive measure.

Finally, in desperation, Shelley called me one day when she was in the midst of a particularly severe attack. She was ready to do "anything," she said, to stop "these blasted blinding migraines from coming back." We were living in different states by then, but I told her how to get started. I warned her, yet again, that this gentle tea takes time to work. She began regularly sipping feverfew tea, sweetened with a spoonful of honey. A few weeks later, Shelley called me again. She was jubilant! She hadn't suffered another migraine, she said, "in ever so long." I rejoiced with her and told her to keep on sipping. She did, for a while. Then her baby was born, she got busy, and forgot about the tea.

One day, she was going about her business when she began to feel the familiar tightening across her forehead. The residual effects of the feverfew had left her system. Shelley told me she began frantically rummaging through the bathroom medicine cabinet looking for something—anything—in the way of a pain reliever. It took many hours before the attack passed. Convinced, she went back to her feverfew tea. No more migraines.

Then Shelley decided to run a little "scientific study" of her own. She wanted to find out for herself if what the scientists call the "placebo effect" was involved. In a true double-blind study, one group is given the active substance, while another group (the control) is given a placebo, or inert substance. No one knows who is taking the active substance, and a few people taking the placebo always report results. If certain people expect a pill to work, placebo or not, it will. Call it the power of suggestion.

Shelley stopped taking feverfew tea. She wanted to find out if the tea was working for her because she expected it to work—which would mean she was under the influence of the placebo effect—or whether the tea was really warding off the migraines she had suffered for so long. Within weeks, she had her answer. She came down with a blinding migraine.

This experience is what turned Shelley into a true believer. In the ensuing years, she has done a lot of research into the old ways. We compare notes now. I can't tell you how gratifying it is to me that she's found the healing teas of help now that she's raising a family of her own. Incidentally, my sister, who suffers from arthritis in both knees, also swears by feverfew. You'll learn all about it in Chapter 6, A Selection of Natural Medicinals.

The healing teas exhibit such a wide range of properties that there's one for just about every ailment under the sun. When my children were small, and even after they were grown, I turned first to propolis tea as a remedy for infections. Garnered from beehives, propolis is the most powerful natural antimicrobial on the planet. It is especially useful against a sore throat. Mahuang, an ancient Chinese herb known on this side of the ocean as ephedra (the forerunner of ephedrine compounds) is a marvellous decongestant. Ginger root sweetens a roiling stomach, calms nausea, and often prevents vomiting. Licorice gives ginger a pleasant boost. Angelica and valerian relieve pain. Chamomile is a mild sedative. Goldenseal, echinacea, and ginseng are strengthening herbs that support the defensive systems of the body. They are useful against all conditions. There are many more. In this book, you'll learn about those I consider the best of the bunch.

Do be aware that healing is often a balancing act. It seems to me that modern medicine has reached a point where it's necessary to balance the beneficial action of some of the more potent drugs against the possibility of real injury due to their sometimes toxic effects. Although there doesn't seem any way around it, this precarious balance can put a patient in harm's way.

By the same token, anyone with a modicum of common sense is faced with the same need for balanced health care. Knowing when to take advantage of modern medicine and when to practice a little self-care health-care is a real balancing act. The healing teas reviewed in this book can be of enormous help. They are not for indiscriminate use and must be taken with appropriately thoughtful and informed care. But, if they are used wisely, I believe healing teas can be as helpful to you and your family as they have been to me and mine.

Part I
Using Teas

. . . and the leaves of the tree were for the healing of nations.

Revelations 22:2

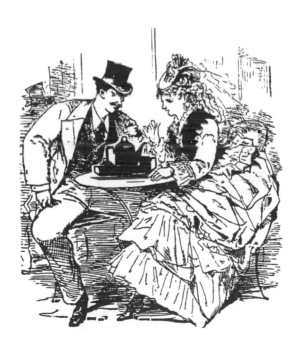

1

Traditional Sipping Teas

Although coffee has come to be the beverage of choice on this side of the ocean, more people around the world drink tea than any other beverage, except water. Entire populations that occupy vast areas of the planet—including Asia, India, Malaysia, the British Isles, the Middle Eastern countries, Africa, and all of the former Soviet Union—start their morning with a steaming cup of tea. In these countries, taking tea throughout the day is common and, in many households, the kettle is always simmering. Tea time is always a pleasant break, a time to socialize if you're with friends, a time to relax if you're alone. Whatever worry may arise, a hot "cuppa" is the answer for many people.

Whether it's "tea for two" by the hearth or a high tea for twenty, there's an undeniable mystique surrounding the simple act of taking tea. The very act of brewing and serving tea to one special someone—or a group you want to impress—turns the interlude into a social occasion. Taking tea can be simple or sophisticated, romantic or urbane, cozy or formal.

In many households, exotic tea blends have taken the place of wine. Where once a bottle of fine old wine was dusted off and decanted with pride, many modern sophisticates now take delight in offering a personally selected tea to guests.

WHAT IS TEA?

Generally speaking, tea is a beverage made by steeping leaves in boiling water. The common tea plant is the evergreen shrub *Camellia sinensis*. Traditionally, tea is prepared from its dried young leaves and leaf buds. Although China is credited with introducing tea to the world, the evergreen tea plant is native to southern China, Assam, Burma, and Cambodia. Assam is a tiny state northeast of India. You'll find it south of China and Bhrutan, tucked between Burma and Pakistan. In any discussion of tea, Assam is important. The Assam variety of *Camellia sinensis* is a very important player in the world of tea.

Although there are an infinite number of hybrids, the three main varieties of the tea plant are China, Assam, and Cambodia. For the moment, forget about the "tiny little tea leaves" of advertising fame and prepare for a surprise. Mature tea leaves range in size from one-and-a-half inches to an amazing ten inches in length.

It's the young leaves that are harvested. In fact, no matter what the variety, the shoot plucked includes the two youngest tea leaves on the stem and a small bud. Because of the need to be so selective, tea is still harvested by hand. Only a trained eye can do this work.

The China variation of *Camellia sinensis* is a many-stemmed bush that reaches a height of nine feet. This tea plant doesn't mind cold temperatures and has a very long lifespan. A healthy China tea bush keeps producing for around one hundred years. When the bush is grown in warmer climes, Darjeeling (India) and Sri Lanka, it's a real money-maker, sending forth tender new shoots twice yearly. It even produces full-flavored leaves in what is called the "second flush."

Assam is the "tea tree." This variety of *Camellia sinensis* grows from twenty to sixty feet high. With expert pruning and regular plucking, it produces for forty years. Tea planters recognize five main subvarieties of Assam teas. For example, there are tender light leaves, less tender dark leaves, the hardy Manipuri (Indian) and Burma varieties, and the very large-leaved Lushai types, grown only in the Lushai hills between India and Burma. The golden-tipped teas produced by dark-leaved Assams during their second flush are considered particularly fine.

The Cambodia variety is also a tree. It attains about sixteen feet in height, but is not a major factor in tea production. Cambodia varieties have mated and married with the other varieties of *Camellia sinensis* on their own.

Unless you are a tea connoisseur, you may be surprised to learn that teas come to us today from such far-flung places as China, Formosa, Japan, India, Sri Lanka, Indonesia, Africa, New Guinea, Taiwan, South America, and Russia. Every single one of these teas is a variety of *Camellia sinensis*. If there is only one tea plant, and that's all there is, how is it that different teas have different tastes? It depends on how the leaves are treated after harvest.

PROCESSING TEA

In spite of the number of countries growing tea and the many blends and brands available, there are only three basic types of *Camellia sinensis*: green, black, and oolong. The difference is in the fermenting. As applied to tea, "fermented" does not signify that tea has been turned into an alcoholic beverage. The light fermentation process undergone by tea leaves refers instead to the enzymatic changes occurring during processing.

Green tea is unfermented; oolong is partially fermented; and black tea is fully fermented. It's the processing that makes all the difference. And, as you'll soon see, not much has changed over the centuries.

Green tea is still the favorite in China, Taiwan, and Japan. In days of old, the freshly plucked leaves were heated in an iron pan for a few minutes to "wither" them, thereby reducing the moisture content. When the leaves turned yellow from the heat, they were taken off the fire, cooled slightly, rolled by hand, and pan-roasted again and again, turning first an olive green shade and finally developing a greenish-blue hue. At this point, the processing was complete and the green tea was ready for brewing. Green tea typically steeps into a mild, slightly bitter, pale greenish-yellow beverage.

Oolong tea comes from a special variety of the China tea plant known as chesima. That's what gives oolong its unique flavor. Oolong brews are slightly bitter and can be brown or amber. The Chinese call these teas wu-lung, which translates to "black dragon." These leaves are processed much the same as China black tea, but more lightly. If you are a fan of oolong, perhaps you particularly enjoy the faint hint of jasmine that is often added to this delightful leaf during processing.

Black tea yields an amber-colored, full-flavored liquid without bitterness. Fully ninety percent of the international trade consists of black tea, in spite of the scads of varieties and blends of tea that abound. Both orange pekoe and pekoe are black teas. The term *pek-ho* is Chinese for "white hair" or "down" and refers to the golden-tipped Assam teas I told you about earlier. Orange pekoe is made from the very young top leaves and traditionally comes from India or Sri Lanka. Pekoe comes from India, Java, or Sri Lanka and is made from leaves even smaller than those characteristically used for orange pekoe.

Another favorite tea that is as popular in the United States as it is in Great Britain, where it originated, is Earl Grey. The formula for this blend is said to have been given to the British earl by a Chinese mandarin. It may surprise you to learn that today there are nine Earl Gray blends, each distinctive, each just a bit different from all the others. Traditional Earl Grey, called Earl Grey Imperial, is a blend of three black teas. The perfume and distinctive taste come from the oil of bergamot that's added during processing. The bergamot tree (*Citrus bergamia*) produces a small citrus fruit. It's the rind that yields the oily essence used in Earl Grey tea.

Of the breakfast teas, English Breakfast is probably the most requested. A blend of small-leafed Ceylon and Indian teas, it's one of the most popular blends in the United States. The rich malty taste of Irish Breakfast comes from the Assam tea leaves of this famed region of India. Those who prefer a heartier brew order Irish Breakfast.

Turning tea leaves into black tea remains a lengthy process. Here's how the ancients did it.

Then as now, the leaves were plucked by hand on a clear day after the dew had dried. The harvest was then laid out in a single layer and exposed to sunlight and air for at least an hour. Next, the leaves were lightly rolled by hand, bruising them and causing a red color to develop. Then they were "withered" in an iron pan, cooled, rolled, and pan-roasted several more times. The final step consisted of further drying. Centuries ago, the leaves were layered in a basket and toasted over a charcoal fire. When cool, the leaves were ready for brewing. Today, about the only part of tea processing that's still done by hand is the plucking. All the rest—from fermenting to air-drying to withering to rolling to the final roasting—has been mechanized.

Once drying is complete, the tea is still not ready to go to market. Remember, there's a big difference in the size of tea leaves, depending on the variety of the tea plant. For example, it takes about 2,000 freshly plucked China tea leaves to make up one pound. But 2,000 freshly harvested Assam leaves weigh in at around two pounds. The leaves must be cut or shredded into tiny particles of roughly uniform size. That's why, if you have your tea leaves read, you won't find one recognizable leaf in the bottom of your teacup.

The shredding process also facilitates blending. According to the Lipton Tea Company, the famous "brisk" Lipton flavor that's been popular in the United States ever since Sir Thomas Lipton set up shop in 1898 comes from a blend of twenty to sixty quality tea varieties.

Walk into a tea shop sometime where loose teas are dispensed by the ounce. You'll often find a bewildering variety of blended teas displayed in glass jars or large tins. Inhale deeply. The heady mingling of scents is almost intoxicating. You're sure to find a leaf to your taste.

THE COMPOSITION OF TEA

When freshly plucked, the tender tea shoot—two young leaves and a bud—is about 77 percent water and 23 percent solids. At least half of the solid matter, consisting mainly of crude fiber, won't dissolve in water. The soluble portion consists of amino acids, caffeine, sugars, vitamins, and organic acids.

A brewed cup of tea contains a moderate amount of caffeine, volatile oils, tannin, and several B-complex vitamins. The flavor of tea is produced by its volatile (rapidly evaporating) oils, while the astringency and color come from the tannin. No matter what tea or blend you favor, it will take a full five minutes of steeping to develop full, rich flavor.

Unless you add sugar and milk, a cup of tea contains only four calories. With the addition of a splash of milk and a lump of sugar, the calorie count will jump to about forty. In Great Britain, where most tea-drinkers sip six cups of milky sugared tea per day, tea consumption adds 240 calories to the average adult's daily diet.

And, surprise, those six cups provide about 10 percent of the RDA for the B-complex vitamins.

Did you ever wonder just how in the world the idea of dropping some leaves into hot water and drinking the result came about? It's rather odd, when you think of it. Actually, the custom of sipping tea began more than four thousand years ago in ancient China.

A WALK THROUGH HISTORY

The earliest recorded mention of tea as a beverage comes to us across the ages in the form of a Chinese scroll brushed in 350 A.D. by a scholar named Lu Yu. This old parchment is named *The Classic of Tea*. In this work, Lu Yu explains the cultivation, processing, and use of tea, then the national beverage of China. Blends were many, even so long ago. Lu Yu says there are "a thousand and ten thousand teas." This ancient scholar also reveals that the brewing of the very first cup of tea was an accident.

It seems that in 2737 B.C., the Chinese Emperor Shen-Nung was boiling some water, a common method of purification even way back then, when some young leaves from a wild tea bush blew unnoticed into the pot. He covered the pot and put it to one side. When Shen-Nung poured the liquid into his cup, he noticed the pale amber color, sniffed the pleasing aroma, and finally took a sip. He found the taste of the steeped leaves very refreshing. Being ever anxious to please their Emperor, the members of the royal court began steeping tea leaves in their boiled drinking water as well. Following that small beginning, China had tea all to itself for around three thousand years.

The Japanese Tea Tradition

Buddhist monks introduced the pleasant practice of drinking tea to Japan around 800 A.D. and assisted in the early cultivation of tea bushes in that country. The Japanese called tea, "the froth of Jade, the elixir of morality." Old pharmacopoeias indicate that for five hundred years, tea was believed to be a medicinal drink. During the fifth century, the Japanese raised tea-drinking to the status of a fine art. The Japanese tea ceremony, called *cha-no-yu*, is very elaborate and of great social and religious significance. The bitter green tea favored by many Japanese is whisked into a pale green froth with a special split bamboo instrument with many fine fronds. The tearoom, known as the *cha-shitsu*, is designed so that the participants must enter on their knees, thereby beginning the ritual with humility.

The ceremony began as a social gathering of friends who drank tea while discussing the aesthetic merits of the elegant and typically spare Japanese art, beautifully brushed calligraphy, and artful flower arrangements. The display of art is usually placed in an alcove, known as the *toko-no-ma*. Often the tea utensils themselves, carefully selected by the tea master for their beauty, are objects of special praise and quiet appreciation.

In the twelfth century, Zen monks sipped tea to keep awake during long meditation periods. They were unaware that the caffeine content was the stimulating factor, but it worked just the same. As time went on, the tea ceremony evolved into a part of a Zen ritual honoring the first patriarch, Bodhidharma.

The tea ceremony underwent further refinement in the sixteenth century court of Toyotomi Hideyoshi, a military dictator who ruled Japan. A member of Hideyoshi's court, Sen Rikyu, was considered a man of aesthetic nature. He was the courtier responsible for the *wabi*-style ceremony, still popular in Japan today. *Wabi*, which means "simplicity," "quiet," and "absence of ornament," remains the very embodiment of this gracious ritual. *Wabi* tea masters prefer simple utensils and strive for a serene atmosphere where nothing unpleasant is permitted to intrude.

In *Chado, The Japanese Way of Tea*, author Soshitsu Sen describes the tea ceremony, which he calls "The Path to Serenity," in these words:

> In the practice of tea, a sanctuary is created where one can take solace in the tranquility of spirit. The utensils are carefully selected and, like the tearoom and garden path, they are cleansed; the writing of a man of virtue is hung in the tokonoma [alcove] and flowers picked that very morning are placed beneath it. The light is natural, but dim and diffused, casting no shadow, and the kettle simmers over the glowing charcoal embers.
>
> The setting thus created is conducive to reflection and introspection. Making tea for oneself in such a setting is sublime. Here, man, nature and the spirit are brought together through the preparation and drinking of tea.

And so it is. If you have never enjoyed this beautifully serene way of experiencing the taking of tea, it will be worth your while to search out a Japanese tea garden where the old ceremony is still practiced. You'll be transported to another realm, another way of life, and come away refreshed, reflective, and just a little bit dreamy.

The Tea Traders

The use of tea spread gradually from all of Asia to the rest of the world. It was carried overland to Russia, but it was the sixteenth century explorers and traders of the Netherlands, France, Portugal, and Britain, with their flying clipper ships, who started the craze for tea in Europe when they brought some of the delicate leaves to their home countries.

Incidentally, the seamen who drank tea suffered far less from amoebic dysentery, a huge problem back then, than did the sailors who drank brackish water right out of the water barrel. Undoubtedly, boiling the water for tea helped kill the "bugs" and effectively sterilized it. Very soon, the exotic oriental beverage the seafaring traders called "t'e" became a hit with the members of the royal court.

It is said that England's Queen Elizabeth I so enjoyed tea that she took it with her morning meal, instead of the more customary ale. The royal physicians who watched over the health of King Louis XIV of France claimed that specially brewed tea soothed and relieved the King's royal headaches. However, taking tea was still a rarity.

The custom of taking tea really took hold when Catherine of Portugal came to London to marry Charles II in 1662. Her dowry included the port of Tangier, which became the tip of the British Empire in Africa, and the island of Bombay, which Charles promptly leased to the newly founded East India Company for 10 pounds sterling per year. Catherine brought something else with her that has become one of the enduring symbols of British life: a chest of her favorite drink—tea.

As the craze for tea grew, the trade between the British Isles and China expanded dramatically. The British established trading centers in Canton and brokered all the tea that came into Europe. When the British East India Company, founded in 1715, lost its monoply on tea in the mid-1800s, the Brits began to search for other sources.

This was when India, still a part of the British Empire, went into the tea business. Shoots of the wild tea growing naturally in Assam began to be cultivated and the industry grew. When the first batch of Indian tea hit the market, it was an immediate success.

The teas of Sri Lanka, formerly Ceylon, were—and are—considered particularly fine. By the way, the teas of Ceylon were so highly regarded, you'll still see Ceylon (not Sri Lanka) listed as the source on tea blends today. This large island at the tip of India originally produced coffee beans, not tea leaves. It wasn't until the coffee plantations of Ceylon fell prey to disease that the planters turned to tea. With India and Ceylon both producing fine teas, the British East India Company continued to be a strong factor in tea exports.

Nonetheless, in spite of the success of the teas of India and Ceylon, China was still the major producer. In 1886, China exported 170 million pounds of tea to Britain. That was over half of the 300 million pounds the Chinese produced. India, the latecomer to the game, produced 90 million pounds.

High Tea

When royalty and the upper classes took to serving four o'clock tea, or "high tea," elaborate sets known as tea services came into being. A typical tea service of the 1800s was handmade of silver and included both tea and coffee pots, milk and cream pitchers, a pair of tea caddies, a sugar bowl with tongs, teaspoons and a small tray to lay them out on, a tea strainer, mote spoons (with tiny bowls and long skinny handles) used to clear leaves from the teapot's spout, and cups and saucers all arranged on a huge tray.

The urn containing the hot water for brewing was placed on a separate stand. Because the urns were large, elaborate, and very heavy, most rested in a swinging cradle so that "milady" did not need to struggle to lift the weight when serving her guests.

Ladies kept their very expensive supply of tea (and equally expensive sugar) under lock and key. By today's standards, the price paid for China tea in the mid-1600s topped out at around

$2,600 per pound. In fact, the cost of tea was equal to the prices nobles paid for gems and baubles for their ladies. One famous jewelry store in Edinburgh sold tea right alongside the precious jewels.

Tea time also meant refreshments, of course. The typically rich high tea would include both "sweets" and "savouries." The menu might include tiny meat pies and sausages alongside dainty crustless sandwiches of cucumber and watercress, plus scones, fresh strawberries, a bowl of clotted cream, biscuits, lemon curd, petit fours, tarts, and small cakes of various flavors.

Considering the price the nobles paid for tea, you might well wonder how the common folk were able to afford it. Although it was Queen Catherine who introduced tea to the court, the experts say smugglers were the ones who brought tea to the masses—not the fine brews royalty enjoyed, of course. The smugglers brought in tea, and unscrupulous merchants bought a bit on the sly. The merchants then adulterated the tea heavily with bark, leaves from other plants, and probably anything else they could get away with.

It didn't take long before tea became the national drink of Great Britain. A family tea might consist of nothing more than bread and butter sandwiches, or a plate of toast and bowl of homemade jam, with the tea served by the mother of the house from a kettle on the stove. But, no matter how simple or elaborate the service, no one ever had to leave the tea table hungry.

The American Colonies

By the eighteenth century, tea was as popular in Britain as it was in the Far East. When British citizens emigrated to the New World, they brought tea cuttings with them, but the climate was inhospitable to the plants. Nonetheless, the transplanted British settlers were accustomed to taking tea and were not prepared to give it up, so the leaves had to be transported by ship.

In 1767, the British king levied a tax on tea. The colonists grumbled and protested without effect. Finally, in 1773, the "boys" got together and threw an entire shipment of precious tea into Boston harbor. Every school child knows that the royal tax on tea, which sparked the Boston Tea Party, was a contributing factor to the Revolutionary War.

Tea contributed to the creation of the United States, and the

United States, in turn, made contributions to the tea industry. Three innovations in tea service and tea packaging came into being in the United States. In the early 1900s, a New York tea merchant by the name of Thomas Sullivan packaged individual samples of his teas in small silk bags. His customers were enchanted with this easy way to brew a single cup of tea, and the first tea bags were born. Iced tea, a summer staple in many households today, was the inspiration of Richard Blechynden, who had a tea stand at the St. Louis Fair in 1904. Because the weather was hot and no one wanted a hot beverage, Blechynden poured freshly brewed tea over ice. It was an immediate sensation. Instant tea is an American invention, too; it was first marketed in 1948.

TEA FOR TASTE

Most traditional tea drinkers drink tea simply because they find the taste pleasing. In this country, the beverage of choice is usually coffee or tea. No one is born with a yen for coffee, tea, or alcoholic spirits. If you're a tea- or coffee- or wine-drinker, think back. I'll bet you made a face as you took your first sip. The delight we come to take in a particular libation grows over time. Tea, like coffee or wine, is an acquired taste.

In France and Italy, it's customary to give young people heavily watered-down wine with their supper. I have a friend who told me she grew up on sugared "coffee-milk." I had a similar introduction to tea. The first cup of tea I was allowed was well-sugared and contained more milk than tea. It was my mother's English heritage, I suppose, that made tea the beverage of choice in our household.

I take my tea "straight" now, but I'm sure it was that first sugary-milky sip that seduced me and started me on my lifelong love of tea. Today, I take a huge delight in sampling all sorts of teas.

Tastes of the traditional sipping teas range from heavy and hearty, to smoky and rich, to bitter and sharp, to pale and light, almost sweet. If you're a coffee drinker, two teas—the traditional sipping tea Assam and an herbal tea blended of roasted grains—come to mind. Either can satisfy the most discriminating dyed-in-the-wool coffee hound.

It's difficult to describe a taste, but there are certain words commonly used to describe a tea blend that conjure up a particular flavor. Table 1.1 reflects a selection of teas distributed by several tea companies. Take a look. If you don't drink tea, you might discover a blend that captures your imagination and decide to give it a try. If you already love tea, you might find the description of a mouth-watering blend that's new to you.

HERB TEAS

Herbal teas are brewed from plants valued for their aroma, taste, and seasoning characteristics as well as for their ability to cause certain subtle changes in body chemistry. Herbs were brewed into healing teas long before they were taken purely for enjoyment. (The medicinal uses of herbs are discussed extensively in Chapter 6.) Today, some herb teas have crossed the borderline between medicine and beverage. That happened when the term "herb tea" was broadened to encompass those delicious blends that include fruits, berries, spices, and other pleasing ingredients. Now, with something for everyone, herb teas are as mainstream as sipping teas.

In the last twenty-five years, a bewildering variety of herbal brews has appeared on the shelves of supermarkets in fancifully decorated and colorful boxes. Many companies now offer what I call "pleasure teas." Blended herbal sipping teas offer a wealth of flavors, depending on their ingredients.

Whether herbs are brewed into healing teas or sipping teas, the plant parts used include the roots, rhizomes (underground, rootlike, horizontal stems), bulbs, barks, flowers, buds, leaves, and stems. You might favor herb teas for their natural goodness and lack of caffeine, or just because the infinite varieties of flavors are immensely appealing. Whether delicate or hearty is "your cup of tea," no one need walk away from a selection of herbal teas without finding some palate-pleasing delicacy.

You might think that these blends all start with a basic herb— chamomile, for example—but that's not always the case.

Chamomile brews into a bland tea and is often used as the base herb in a blend, but there are other popular base ingredients. Rose hips are usually the basic tea in the fruit-flavored blends, and smoothly roasted grains often form the base for the heartier herbal tea blends.

If you're in the market for a new favorite, all that's necessary

Table 1.1 Traditional Sipping Teas

Variety	Taste	Notes of Interest	Body
Assam	Heavy, malty	The "coffee-drinkers" tea	Rich
Ceylon	Bright, mild	Long-lasting aroma	Full
Ceylon Breakfast	Light, flowery	"Golden" orange pekoe blend	Mild
China Rose	Sweet, rose flavor	Blended with rose petals and buds	Light
Darjeeling	Lively, real "tea" taste	Traditional "afternoon" tea	Full
Earl Grey	Lively, with hint of citrus	Three-tea blend, with oil of bergamot	Medium
English Breakfast	Well-rounded, bright, lively	Original 1706 recipe	Full
Irish Breakfast	Rich, robust, pungent	Small leaf Assam blend	Hearty
Jasmine	Light, flowery flavor	Petals are layered in with tea	Medium
Keemun	Full, slightly sweet	Very old Chinese blend	Medium
Lapsang Souchong	Light and smoky	Leaves traditionally smoked over burning rubber	Medium
Lemon	Light, lemony taste	Medium leaf blend with lemon essence	Light
Prince of Wales	The "burgundy" of teas	Exclusively blended of leaves from Anhwei Province	Rich
Pingsuey	Mild, delicate	Uniquely Chinese Hard to find	Medium
Russian	Heavy, sharp	Keemun, Lapsang Souchong blend	Medium
Russian Caravan	Rich, superb brown blend.	China black and Oolong Cherished by old Russian aristocracy	Rich
Yunnan	Brisk, "winey" flavor	An old China-type tea	Light

is to read the label. The list of ingredients reveals the wonders inside each little tea bag. Blended herb teas can be richly fruity with hints of apple, orange, and lemon grass. They can be sweet and spicy with cinnamon, cloves, and more. With one of the mints as the basic ingredient, herb teas become refreshing pick-me-ups. Still other blends invite sleep with the mild flavor of the soothing and calming herbs, like chamomile.

Coffee-drinkers might like the rich blend of roasted grains and selected spices, with carob providing just a hint of chocolate, in

Brewing the Noble Leaf

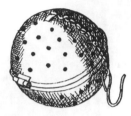

Figure 1.   Tea Ball

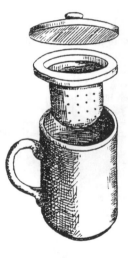

Figure 2.   Tea Mug

Back when tea was so costly that only royalty could afford it, tea was known as the "noble leaf." But you don't have to be "to the manor born" to enjoy tea today. You don't need a fancy tea service either. To brew a single cup, all you need is a china or glass cup and a tea bag. If you favor loose tea, you can use a hinged and perforated stainless steel tea ball (shown in Figure 1). Simply open the ball, put in a spoonful of tea, drop the ball in a cup of freshly boiled water, pop a lid on the cup, and let the tea steep. You'll also find special tea mugs that are fitted with a perforated infuser and have their own lids (as shown in Figure 2).

To my way of thinking, the least satisfactory method of brewing a single cup of loose tea is to use a perforated stainless steel spoon (as shown in Figure 3). The reason why I don't care for these spoons becomes obvious when you realize that the handle protrudes and there's no way to cover the cup so the tea can steep. The best you can do with one of these spoons is stir, and that just won't give you a full-flavored cup of tea.

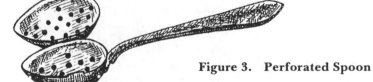

Figure 3.   Perforated Spoon

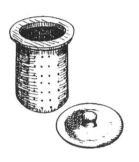

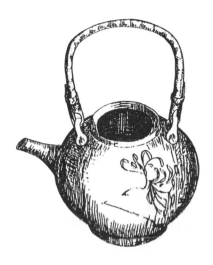

Figure 4.   Tea Pot With Infuser

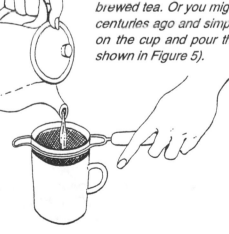

The time-tested method of brewing tea in a pot remains the best. If you don't have a pot, there are several types you might investigate. For example, many teapots come with a perforated infuser designed to hold loose tea (as shown in Figure 4). Others have a built-in strainer at the base of the spout to hold back the wet leaves. Either type of pot, with infuser or strainer, makes it easy to enjoy freshly brewed tea. Or you might do as "milady" did centuries ago and simply rest a tea strainer on the cup and pour the tea through it (as shown in Figure 5).

Figure 5.   Pouring Tea Through a Strainer

The brewing of fine tea is best done in china, glass, or stainless steel. Never steep tea in plastic or aluminum. Don't use an aluminum kettle for boiling water for brewing tea either.

Always fill your teapot with hot water to preheat it. Empty it out only when the brewing water is ready.

Preparing the Brewing Water

Always use fresh bottled water for brewing tea. Tap water contains chemicals that can alter the taste of a brew. Heat water for brewing to the temperatures suggested below, depending on the tea you are using. Never reheat water left in the kettle either. Reheating water results in a flat cup of tea. It may seem terribly odd to give you directions for boiling water, but the correct steeping temperature is critical for certain teas, so please read on.

__Green Teas; Light, Flowery Herbals.__ Steep in water at the first boil. This is when the water first begins to bestir itself. It's restless, but not yet simmering. If you are using a thermometer, water at the first boil should register 160°F. It's better to steep delicate teas a little longer using water at a lower temperature than it is to force the leaves to give up their essence with high temperatures and end up with a bitter brew.

__Oolongs; Semi-fermented Teas; Most Herbal Blends.__ Steep in water at the second boil. This water is dancing and hissing with impatience. There are bubbles rising across the entire surface; it's starting to steam, on the verge of erupting. Water on the second boil will register between 180 and 195°F.

__Heavy Black Teas; Herbals with Roasted Ingredients.__ Steep in water at the third boil. Water at a full, rollicking boil is what's needed to release the full flavors of heavy traditional teas and hearty herb blends. You don't need a thermometer to identify water on the third boil.

When the brewing water is ready, empty the teapot and put a suitable amount of tea into it—one teabag or one rounded teaspoon of loose tea per cup. Add boiling water, cover, and let steep for three to five minutes (three minutes for light flavor; five minutes for full rich flavor). Flavor increases with the length of the steeping period. Some teas produce color quickly, but don't be deceived. You can't judge when a tea is ready solely by color; take a test sip. Full flavor depends on at least three—preferably five—minutes of steeping time.

many of the teas that are marketed as "coffee substitutes." My advice is to enjoy them for what they are. These teas taste too good to "substitute" for anything.

There's a huge selection of delicious herbal sipping teas on the market. If you can't find something you like, you just aren't trying. The varieties of teas and tea blends keep growing. From traditional to herbal, there are so many different flavors to explore that every individual taste can be satisfied.

IT'S TEA TIME

Dawdling over a luscious high tea isn't just for society leaders and ladies any longer. Business men and women and high-powered politicians are now meeting for tea between 2 and 6 P.M. Where business was once traditionally conducted during what came to be known as the "power lunch," tea time is now the venue of choice for the wheeler-dealers. Small tearooms with dainty, lacy napkins have lost their monopoly on tea time. They have been edged out as elegant restaurants and hotels have taken advantage of this latest craze for tea. All around the country, restaurants and hotels are serving tea. Manhattan's most plush waterholes, including the Plaza, the Waldorf-Astoria, the Pierre, and the St. Regis, now feature high teas.

You don't have to negotiate a million-dollar deal to take afternoon tea, you know. If you are not yet an afficionado of tea, visit one of the hotels in your area and enjoy a leisurely high tea served in an elegant setting. While you sample tiny tarts, nibble thin cucumber sandwiches, or munch ripe, red strawberries with clotted cream, you will be enjoying the same type of feast that royalty all over the world finds such an indispensable and relaxing part of the day.

If you order tea in a restaurant, many times you'll be served a teapot full of freshly boiled water, with a selection of individually wrapped tea bags—both traditional and herbal—in a basket so you can choose your favorite. Everywhere you look, more and more people are taking tea.

Tea has always been a popular beverage in this country and is undeniably enjoying a resurgence in popularity. Although coffee has overtaken tea as the national drink, there are those among us who drink nothing but tea, those who switch from coffee to tea midday, and many more who look forward to a steaming cup of their favorite tea, be it green, black, oolong—or herbal—at the end of a long day.

And, if you have discovered the joys of Thai food and have a favorite Thai restaurant, perhaps you have also become a fan of Thai iced tea. Strictly speaking, this tea falls somewhere between traditional and herbal. It is composed of five finely pulverized ingredients, including peanuts and corn, plus three Thai herbals. Thai iced tea is served in a tall glass over crushed ice. The delicious blend is topped off with a liberal splash of sweet cream. Even if you don't like tea, you'll like this sweet and creamy concoction.

SOMETHING FOR EVERYONE

There are just so many sipping teas around that the infinite variety boggles the mind. If you don't see something you like, wait awhile. From traditional to herbal, new tea blends are coming onto the market all the time.

Please pause here and think back for a moment. It all started in 2737 B.C. in China when an errant breeze accidentally blew some tender tea leaves into Shen-Nung's pot of boiling water. There's no way Shen-Nung could have envisioned all the uses for tea—both traditional and medicinal—that have developed in the last 5,000 years.

In the next chapter, I'll give you a look at the ancient healing systems that developed the medicinal brews. Not surprisingly, healing teas originated in China, too.

2

Traditional Healing Teas

W hile sipping teas are taken primarily for the enjoyment they offer, healing teas are taken for the subtle alterations in body chemistry they provide. Healing teas are traditionally brewed from herbs and other natural medicinals found in nature's pharmacy.

Ancient physicians made full and effective use of the natural medicines all around them. Our knowledge today of brewing and applying healing teas has its roots in the old time-tested healing systems.

IN THE BEGINNING

The recorded history of natural medicine and the healing teas dates back over 5,000 years, although medicinal plants were certainly used even earlier. Long before any written records existed, there were healers. For millennia, man has contended with sickness and disease. The healers of primitive times were the priests and priestesses, the shamans and witch doctors, the medicine men and women, those special few who were believed able to commune with the mighty powers of the universe. Ancient healers sang incantations to lure the drifting and sickly spirit back into the body. Egyptian physicians, in a practice called trepanning, cut holes in the skull to let out the evil spirits that carried disease, and petitioned the gods for relief with prayers and chants.

Early man discovered by trial and error which plants were suitable as food sources, and gradually identified those with valuable medicinal qualities. The healing plants were sought after, carefully dried, and stored for use as needed. Somewhere along the way, man also identified the plants that were fatal and used their juices on darts, spears, and arrows to bring death to their enemies.

These were an unsophisticated short-lived people, accustomed to unending hardship. Minor health problems, like aching joints, an infected tooth, constipation, and diarrhea, were accepted as a part of life and ignored, for the most part. Primitive man believed any serious health problem either came from evil spirits that insinuated themselves into the victim, or was terrifying evidence that the victim had offended some powerful god. A wound sustained by a hunter or warrior was washed and dressed with clean leaves, but if an infection developed, it was because the gods so decreed.

Medicinal plants and herbs were used to help the wounded and the seriously sick, but they were administered along with incantations, frenzied dancing, and loud banging of drums. These activities were designed to attract the benevolent intervention of the gods and drive away the evil spirits that brought disease. As the healing teas worked, the patients were comforted by the rituals performed on their behalf by the tribe's medicine man. Patients rested more easily, secure in the thought that the gods had been persuaded to intercede on their behalf. Ancient healers treated both mind and body. They were the original holistic physicians.

EVERYTHING OLD IS NEW AGAIN

I'm going to skip across the centuries for a moment to point out that prevention, long out of favor in Western medicine, is making a comeback. Some health insurance companies are beginning to pay for well-baby checkups, annual physicals, even diet and lifestyle counseling.

The ancient systems of medicine all rely on prevention, first, on balance (inside and out), next, and on treating a particular condition, last. In evaluating and diagnosing a patient, many things are taken into consideration that go beyond the obvious symptoms. In all the ancient healing traditions, the physician takes time to learn everything there is to know about a particular patient that may impact on his health, including his state of mind, the emotions he might be struggling with, any stress (physical or mental) he is laboring under, the foods he eats, the water he drinks, whether he has a sedentary or active lifestyle, even the environment and climate where he lives. Only after all these elements are duly noted and factored in is the treatment regimen laid out and the prescriptions for healing teas dispensed.

Before we discuss the healing teas as they can benefit you today, it will be useful to understand how the oldest medical traditions in the world are practiced. Even today, physicians who are schooled in the ancient healing systems of China and India continue to practice a highly refined form of natural medicine that is completely compatible with the human body. Both approaches rest on the strong foundation of healing teas.

THE ANCIENT TRADITIONS

Chinese healers were—and are—holistic in their approach to healing. The key factor in the Chinese approach to health is harmony or balance. The aim of the Chinese physician is to balance the body's yin and yang. You probably already know that Chinese tradition holds that all things have opposing yet complementary attributes. For example, yin is female and rules the night. Yang is male and rules the day. When balance between yin and yang has been achieved and health and harmony have been restored, there will be a smooth flow of energy—chi—along the patient's internal pathways, known as meridians. Acupuncture points follow the meridians.

In diagnosis, the traditional Chinese physician uses the techniques of looking, listening, smelling, asking, and touching. Internal harmony, or lack of it, shows in a patient's appearance. How many times have you looked in the mirror and thought, "I look terrible. This infection is really getting me down"? Your posture, facial expression, complexion, manner, and spirit are the first clues showing a lack of harmony to the Chinese doctor. Next, your tongue is checked out. In Chinese medicine, as in orthodox medicine, the appearance of your tongue is known as a never-fail indicator of what's going on inside your body. Changes in the appearance of the tongue offer vital clues to the nature of an illness.

The physician will next listen to your breathing, the timber of your voice, and the sounds rumbling around inside your lungs as you cough on command. That's familiar to all of us who grew up with Western medicine, but all the while, the Chinese practitioner is delicately breathing in the scent your body puts forth. He's looking for a "foul" or "pungent" odor, which can provide yet more clues to the nature of illness.

Just as an orthodox physician takes a case history before treating a new patient, the Chinese physician asks about your medical and family history, but he won't stop there. He'll list symptoms and question you closely about your lifestyle. He might want to know what you had for lunch and what your favorite foods are, if you have a strong appetite or couldn't care less what time dinner is served, whether you perspire a lot or a little, how much water you drink and what degree of thirst you have, how many times a day you visit the bathroom, even whether you are sensitive to heat or cold. By the time this intimate question-session is over, you'll just about be convinced the doctor either wants to be your best friend or is a spy whose mission is to report all your little peccadillos to your mother.

Next comes touching. Trained fingers will travel the meridians of your body, feeling for any sore points and pausing to investigate any lumps or bumps. By far, the most important diagnostic tool in Chinese medicine is the taking of the pulse. You've probably had your pulse taken, but, unless your health-care provider is schooled in the ancient arts, never like this: First of all, the doctor will feel for your pulse at three different positions on each wrist. All told, the traditional Chinese healer is trained in evaluating the meaning of twenty-eight different pulses. Each pulse point corresponds to and reveals the condition of different areas of the body. The Doctrine of the Pulse is such an important part of Chinese medicine that many patients still say, "I'm going to have my pulse felt," when a doctor's visit is on the agenda.

Only after the diagnosis is complete will a treatment plan be laid out. Treatment can consist of any or all of the time-tested ancient therapies, including acupuncture, massage, moxibustion, exercise, diet, and herbal remedies. A Chinese physican will write out a prescription, just as an orthodox physician does. The only difference is that you'll take this script for a healing tea to a Chinese pharmacy to have it filled.

The typical Chinese herb shop contains a vast array of herbs stored in tightly-closed glass jars, some mysterious closed drawers, and exotic-looking chests full of the more costly ingredients. Unless you can read Chinese, don't even try to figure out what the glass jars contain. If something looks like the proverbial "eye of newt" from a witch's brew, don't worry. The pharmacist knows what he's doing.

Picture this: First, a clean square of parchment is laid out. Next, the pharmacist expertly weighs the prescribed amounts of the various herbs—almost all Chinese prescriptions are complex, combination remedies—one after the other. After each ingredient is weighed, the raw herb goes onto the parchment in a little heap. By the time the prescription is filled, the paper is crowded and you're beginning to wonder how in the world you're going to brew a tea out of all those odd-sized buds, dried leaves, chunks of bark, and what looks like dry yellow sticks. Don't disgrace yourself by asking. The pharmacist next takes the whole kit and kaboodle, grinds it into a smooth powder, slides the powder into a Ziploc plastic bag (sorry, tradition loses out to modern convenience) and you're on your way with a 5,000-year-old remedy that is just as effective today as it was when it was first formulated.

The first written instructions for brewing healing teas date back to ancient China and the legendary Fu Hsi, who lived almost 3,000 years before the Christian era began. Shen-Nung, who died in 2698 B.C. continued the tradition, followed by Huang Ti, who departed this world in 2598 B.C. The most famous of the old Chinese emperors who left written works pertaining to medical matters has to be Huang-di, the Yellow Emperor. He is said to be the author of the *Nei Ching*, a materia medica of internal medicine that dates back 2,000 years. The *Mo Ching* or Pulse Classic came along much later in 300 A.D.

The most comprehensive of the old herbal instruction manuals is the *Pen-ts-ao kang-mu*, better known as the *Great Pharmacopoeia*, put together by the scholar Li Shih-chen (1552–1578). His work, still authoritative today, is a compilation of all previous materia medica. The *Great Pharmacopoeia*, totaling fifty-two volumes, is a work worthy of a long lifetime, yet Li Shih-chen died at the age of twenty-six.

This work includes the Doctrine of Signatures, which holds that the shape of plants and roots, or the marks appearing naturally on them, indicates how man should use them. For example, ginseng root looks very much like a human figure, suggesting its use as an all-over body tonic. The flower of the lobelia plant is shaped rather like a stomach, indicating its emetic qualities. Goldenseal has a greenish-yellow root, which suggests its use in jaundice and infections of all types. Whether you hold with the Doctrine of Signatures or think it nothing more than a charming myth from long ago, it's interesting to know that the preceding effects have all been confirmed in recent research. However, there's one myth that doesn't hold up.

Picture a rhino horn, and you'll understand why the Doctrine of Signatures assigned this appendage aphrodisiacal properties. Incidentally, rhino horn isn't horn at all. It's a tightly twisted mass of keratin, a protein found in hair. And it's not an aphrodisiac either.

Many of the Chinese brews still in use provide the same medicinal ingredients used in today's drugs. For example, mahuang of the genus *Ephedra*, has been used in Chinese medicine for at least 4,000 years. Ephedrine, extracted from mahuang, has migrated into Western medicine and is used to treat asthma and other forms of respiratory distress. It is also an ingredient in many over-the-counter (OTC) decongestants.

Chinese healers of old prescribed iron for anemia, used castor oil and Chinese rhubarb to relieve constipation and purge the body, administered kaolin (think Kaopectate) to treat diarrhea, used camphor as an antiseptic, and employed chaulmoogra oil to treat leprosy back when most civilizations were crying, "Unclean," and running away from victims of this horrifying condition. The Chinese also used rauwolfia to treat high blood pressure and certain nervous conditions centuries before Western medicine caught on, extracted reserpine, and found it worked wonderfully well.

The common foxglove, from which the cardiac drug digitalis is extracted, has been "on the books" so long in Chinese medicine that it appears in the *Nei Ching*. This plant also offers verodoxin, a substance that potentiates digitalis so well that smaller doses are required to achieve the desired effect.

Still, no matter how well the medicinals worked, the main aim of the ancients was to prevent an illness from taking hold. Legend has it that ancient Chinese healers were paid a monthly fee to keep their patients well. They prescribed strengthening health-building herbal teas, designed individual diet plans, laid out programs of exercise, and generally mandated a healthy lifestyle. These doctors made "house calls," too. They practically hovered over their clients, sympathized with all their problems, and continually encouraged them to live healthfully.

Here's the catch. If a client fell ill, the doctor's monthly fee stopped until the patient was completely well. Needless to say, this "incentive pay plan" was powerful motivation to practice the finest, most meticulous preventive medicine ever known. And when a servant came crying, "Learned physician, my master is ill in his bed," the doctor grabbed his herbs and tools of the trade, hastened to his client's bedside, brewed healing teas on the spot, and stayed until the patient was up and around again. Only then was the physician's monthly stipend due and payable again.

The Chinese physician of old did have an escape hatch, however. If a client refused to follow his carefully planned regimen for health, the doctor was free to drop him from his list of clients.

Unless your health-care provider is a licensed practitioner of Chinese medicine, you'll find it difficult to take advantage of this centuries-old healing tradition today. Chinese herbal remedies are very complex formulations. You can't walk into a true Chinese pharmacy, pick and choose several ingredients, and have the raw herbs ground to order. You can, however, brew some simple teas with the old time-tested Chinese herbs. I'll tell you about the best Chinese herbs in Part II, Selecting Teas.

India

Most authorities agree that the Chinese were first to use herbs and healing teas medicinally, although some argue it was actually the holy men of India who carried the ancient knowledge to China. Whenever you compare the two most ancient systems of medicine in the world, there's no denying they share similarities. A very old text expresses the Hindu belief in preventive medicine this way: "Heyam dukham anagatam," which means "Avert the danger which has not yet come." Ayur-Ved is an ancient Hindu system of medicine that goes back to the second millennium B.C. The word comes from two Sanskrit roots: *Ayus* or "life," and *Veda*, which translates to "knowledge" or "science." Thus, the literal meaning of Ayur-Ved is the "science of life."

As in Chinese medicine, the techniques practiced in the healing tradition of Ayurvedic medicine are holistic, meaning that both the mind and body are treated at the same time. There's a lot of crossover in the ancient healing traditions. For example, the Doctrine of the Pulse—a diagnostic tool used to detect a subtle imbalance in the body—is common to both Chinese and Ayurvedic tradition, although the techniques vary somewhat.

When you visit the *vaidya*, or Ayur-Ved physician, you will be the object of a most careful diagnosis. In this healing system, relying both on observation and questioning, the physician will first establish your particular *dosha*, or mind-body type. Centuries of experience have shown that the doshas predominating in the mind-body system give rise to specific and quite different emotional, mental, and physical tendencies. Each person is born with a unique psycho-physiological profile that is reflected in his dosha.

Although there is infinite individual variety and the vaidya will consider many shadings, here's a general run-down on the main doshas: *Vata* types are slender, active and energetic, vivacious, enthusiastic, imaginative, and quick. *Pitta* types generally have a medium build, enjoy a strong metabolism and good digestion, have sharp intellect, and speak well, but tend to be irritable. *Kapha* types gain weight easily, are heavily built, have great stamina and physical endurance, maintain a slow pace, and have a tranquil personality.

The aim of the techniques practiced in Ayur-Ved is to address any imbalances, take appropriate measures to restore balance, and, finally, identify any problems to which a person may be prone. A preventive health program will be designed using healing teas to "avert the danger which has not yet come."

Old Ayurvedic manuscripts set forth detailed listings of specific herbal brews for the treatment of many medical conditions. The principal Ayurvedic text, the Charaka Samhita, lists herbal preparations called *rasayana* that promise "longevity, memory, intelligence, freedom from disorders, youthful age, excellence of luster, complexion and voice, optimum strength of physique and sense organs, successful words, respectability and brilliance."

In India today, people routinely visit a vaidya who prescribes the medicinal herbal compounds they need to brew healing teas. Some of the most ancient rasayanas have been recreated in their purest forms. One very complex herbal compound—Amrit Nectar—requires twenty-two pounds of fruits and herbs to produce one pound of nectar. This authentic Ayur-Ved formula contains, among other things, *amalaki* (Indian gooseberry), *ghee* (clarified butter), *Gokarna* (butterfly pea), *vriddha-daraka* (elephant creeper), *brahmi* (Indian pennywort), *brihat-upa-unchika* (cardamom), heart-leaved moonseed, black musale, Indian globe thistle, and raw sugar. Quite obviously, there's no way to prepare authentic Amrit Nectar at home.

In Sanskrit, *amrit* means "deathless." Hence, the Amrit Nectar rasayana is said to be "the ambrosial drink that confers immortality." In fact, research has shown that Amrit Nectar has the ability to neutralize free radicals better and faster than the antioxidant vitamins that are so much in the news today. Because free radicals are implicated in heart disease, cancer, and accelerated aging, here's yet another instance where science has validated the old wisdom.

Although the necessary ingredients for Ayurvedic teas aren't readily available for home brewing, in Chapter 4, Shopping for Healing Teas, I'll tell you where you can purchase some prepared Ayurvedic tea blends especially designed to complement all three main dosha types.

The Greeks and Romans

Because both Chinese medicine and Ayurvedic healing are still practiced today much as they were centuries ago, tracking the healing systems of both China and India is relatively easy. Moreover, written records of these ancient systems have survived for millennia, including the precise formulas for the brewing and blending of healing teas. Written records also give us access to Greek and Roman healing techniques.

About 370 B.C., the Greek Theophrastus, a pupil of Plato and fellow pupil of Aristotle, published *An Enquiry Into Plants*. This work included a section entitled "The Juices of Plants and the Medicinall Properties of Herbs." Later learned men also relied on herbs. Galen (c 130–200 A.D.), a famed physician of early Greece who prepared his own medicines from his well-stocked apothecary, kept hyoscyamus, opium, squill, and viper toxin on hand. Galen used squill, an onion-like sea vegetable, as an expectorant, heart stimulant, and diuretic. Hyoscyamus, perhaps more familiar to us as the herb henbane, is an ancient sedative with antispasmodic properties. The leaves contain crude scopolamine, still used medically today.

Early in the first century, Pliny the Elder and another Greek physician produced a book listing herbal teas and including hand-colored illustrations of various medicinal plants. This incredible achievement has not survived, but the experts say the vital information contained therein was included in the *Materia Medica* of Pedanius Dioscorides, a Greek physician who served in the Roman army. This extensive work covers plant remedies used in Egypt, Greece, and the Roman empire.

Other Ancient Traditions

It's much more difficult to find a comprehensive history of the herbal brews used in other traditions. It is, however, written that Egyptian physicians of the first and second century A.D. prescribed ipecac to cause vomiting, treated constipation with a tea brewed from senna pods, and used caraway tea to relieve indigestion. Egyptian physicians, as depicted in hieroglyphs dating from the first century A.D., also used peppermint to relieve digestive problems. These prescriptions are still valid, and still familiar, today.

From the *Materia Medica*, a book of medical prescriptions written in the first century B.C., we have learned that Egyptian physicians used verdigris as a medicinal agent. Verdigris, the greenish patina that forms on copper, is a copper compound. We know today that copper potentiates iron absorption, making it a useful adjunct to the diet of an anemic patient. It would appear that the ancients also knew that copper was healthful.

We know for certain that herbs were very important in Biblical times. The Hebrew Torah includes mention of the use of certain bitter herbs at Passover. There are thirty-eight direct references to "herb" or "herbs" in the King James translation of the Holy Bible. In Psalms 104:14, we find the promise, ". . . and herb for the service of man." There are many references that mention specific herbals by name. According to the Bible, frankincense and myrrh were so holy when used as perfumes and annointing oils that they were reserved for the priesthood and forbidden to ordinary citizens.

There are even Bible verses that show the healing power of nature's pharmacy. In Revelations 22:2, we read, ". . . and the leaves of the tree were for the healing of the nations." But my personal favorite, and the passage most often cited to substantiate the God-given medicinal power of herbs, is found in Ezekiel 47:12, ". . . and the leaf thereof for medicine." The medicinal components of a great many herbs are deposited in their leaves, which makes them perfectly suited for brewing into healing teas. I think that's part of God's grand design, not an accident.

It is not surprising that the ancients placed such stock in herbals. Consider that the famous Code of Hammurabi, formulated by one of Babylon's early kings, lists laws under which physicians worked. If you think a doctor hauled into court today and charged with malpractice is in trouble, consider that the law in 1800 B.C. stated: "If the doctor, in opening an abscess, shall kill the patient, his hands shall be cut off." It's no wonder physicians preferred prescribing teas to performing surgery.

The ancient Arabs quickly surpassed their contemporaries in their knowledge of chemistry and in the preparation of medicinal drugs. Distillation, the process of removing impurities and concentrating the essence of a substance by evaporation, was developed by the Arabs centuries ago. Sublimation, a form of purification that reduces a substance to crystalline form, was also an Arabian process. It appears that knowledge about drug preparation and herbs was not always so prevalent in Europe.

EUROPEAN MEDICINE

Although it seems incredible to us today, during the Middle Ages, the worth of a doctor was judged by the *filthiness* of his coat. As far as the public was concerned, the more blood and gore staining his coat, the better the doctor. A dirty coat was evidence of a thriving practice. The professional physician practiced bloodletting and purging and preferred cutting to administering drugs. These practices were in direct contrast to the system used by the traditional healer, who believed in the power of healing teas and preferred a less invasive and more patient approach.

It really wasn't until the Black Death or bubonic plague surfaced in 1348 that Europeans realized the offerings of medical professionals weren't working. No amount of bloodletting and purging, which was supposed to rid the body of disease-causing "ill-humours," stopped the progression of the disease. After one-third of the population of Europe had succumbed to the plague, the public began cautiously (and secretly) to turn once again to the old tried and true remedies of the herbalists. But professional physicians were contemptuous of "old-fashioned" healing teas, and they still held forth as authorities on all matters regarding health.

All that began to change when syphilis surfaced as a major medical problem in the 1500s. It was thought that Columbus' crew had brought syphilis to Europe after voyaging to the West Indies. Unlike the Black Death, syphilis involved suffering of long duration and its victims usually went mad before they died. Because the disease took a while to progress, the physicians had an opportunity to experiment with various "cures." What they finally settled on was mercury, so toxic that it was deadly in itself. Nonetheless, the disease was so feared that patients continued to swallow the "mercury cure."

In 1574, a French physician by the name of Nicholas Monardes published an account advocating the use of sarsaparilla for syphilis. Sarsaparilla was eagerly welcomed as a sure-cure for the dreaded disease. It was widely believed that a disease native to a region could be cured by medicinal plants from the same region. Sarsaparilla, from the New World, would cure the disease because, according to popular belief, syphilis had originated in the New World. It is interesting to note that, much later, clinical studies determined that sarsaparilla is effective in about 90 percent of the cases of acute syphilis and about 50 percent of the cases of chronic syphilis.

A twentieth century book on medieval and renaissance medicine reports that guaiac, another natural medicinal found in the New World, was a cure for syphilis. This bark was called "palo santo" or "holy wood" by the Spaniards.

The first pharmacopoeia with a collection of medicinals and directions for their preparation came from Johann Gutenberg in 1546. Interestingly, the twelfth book printed after the famous Gutenberg Bible, the first secular book ever printed, was *De Agricultura*, written by an Italian named Peter Crescentius.

Gerard's Herbal was published in 1597. Nicholas Culpeper's first book, *The English Physician*, appeared in the early 1600s. This book recommended common English herbs that could be found in many backyard gardens. Many medical books of the time survive, including—incredibly—a Latin language version of an Aztec manuscript that lists many native plants and describes their healing powers. (Just to keep the times in perspective, Shakespeare achieved his first real recognition as a playwright in 1584.)

THE CHANGING FACE OF MEDICINE

In 1617, the Society of Apothecaries was founded in London. Only a member of the society was permitted to keep an apothecary's shop and prepare and sell natural medicinals. The society's bible, the *London Pharmacopoeia*, was published in 1618. It contained standardized formulas for the proper preparation of herbal drugs.

The *London Pharmacopoeia* wasn't available to the masses, but the common man benefited greatly from Nicholas Culpeper's *A Compleat Herbal*, published in 1649. This work is a respected pharmacopoeia from a master herbalist of the times. It is still widely referred to and quoted today.

Don't forget, for many centuries, healers gathered their own medicinals or bought them from locals who grew and harvested them or foraged local fields. Doctors personally compounded the ingredients for the healing teas they dispensed and were jealous of their formulas. When apothecary shops first came onto the scene, the physicians wrote the prescriptions and apothecaries filled them, but the doctor still compounded his own medicines. Using a mortar and pestle, the physician (or his assistant) ground the herbs for teas before they were dispensed to the patient with detailed instructions for use.

In 1841, the Pharmaceutical Society of Great Britain was founded and education and training of pharmacists became mandatory. Apothecary shops dispensed standardized herbal compounds, but this was still the Dark Ages as far as medical practice was concerned.

People did just about anything to stay out of the hospitals, with good reason. Most people who went into a hospital came out feet first. Filth was the great leveler. Although the physicians didn't know it, death often occurred because doctors transferred deadly bacteria from one patient to another as they made their rounds.

Baron Joseph Lister, the famed London surgeon, changed all that in 1865 by demonstrating that antiseptic procedures and basic cleanliness saved lives.

Things were looking up, but it was still "self-care health-care" for the most part. Home-brewed healing teas were a staple in every household. Shops with trained apothecaries were found only in big cities, and published manuscripts were beyond the reach of most persons. However, the methods of brewing medicinal teas were traditionally passed from generation to generation by word of mouth.

THE NEW WORLD

Early American settlers brought their medicinal teas and precious seeds to the new world so the knowledge and skills would not be lost. The colonists learned from the Native Americans about herbs native to North America, and the cycle continued.

An early report of native American herbs was made by an Englishman named Whitaker who wrote home with "good news from Virginia." He included mention of many native plants, including "pine, pitchtrees, soape ashes, cedar, ash, maple and cypress and sassafras, which is called by the inhabitants Winauk, and is a kind of wood of most pleasant and sweet smell, with rare virtues in phisick for the cure of many diseases."

The herbal knowledge of the Native Americans was welcomed by the early Colonists. Obviously dependent on local plants for their remedies, colonists had a healthy respect for native vegetation. In 1621, an Englishman wrote:

> We are told that the Indians and themselves are falling into a contagious disease, of which Phisitians [physicians] could give no reason or remedy, yet they were all in a short space restored to their health merely by drinking water; in which Saxifrage [sassafras] was infused and boyled; which was discovered to them by the natives; and wee justly entertain beliefe that many excellent medicines either for conservation of Nature in her vigour or restauration in her decadence may be communicated unto us . . .

Another publication that gives insight into early Colonial medicine was written by John Josselyn in 1672. This pamphlet was entitled *New England Rarities Discovered . . . and Chyrurgical remedies wherewith the natives constantly used to cure their distempers, wounds and sores.* The experts say authoritative research shows that, all told, Native American remedies added fifty-nine drugs to the modern pharmacopoeia.

The Shaker Apothecaries

As the colonies became the American nation, cities began to develop in the late eighteenth and early nineteenth centuries. Unless they had an abundant kitchen garden, most people had no access to fresh herbs. They were dependent on the local apothecary shop. The shop, in turn, was dependent on locals who combed the woods, and farmers who raided their own gardens for the healing herbs.

The Shakers, members of the Church of the United Society of Believers, saw the need and filled it. In effect, as the first "pharmaceutical company" on these shores, the Shakers were the fore runners of the giant drug companies. They pioneered the mass production and marketing of herbal medicinals. A shaker "apothecary" is shown in Figure 2.1.

In the 1820s, the Shakers seeded their first "physic garden" in New York. History records that by 1857, in one season alone, 75 tons of medical plants were grown, dried, pressed, packed, and shipped to customers all over the young nation, as well as abroad

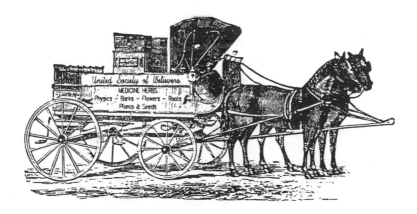

Figure 2.1 Shaker Apothecary Wagon

to London and even as far as Australia. Just prior to the outbreak of the Civil War, the Shaker apothecary included an extensive list totalling 354 kinds of medicinal plants, barks, roots, seeds, and flowers. The Shakers earned a reputation for effective, reasonably priced medicinals and honest dealings.

Home treatment of many ills was a way of life during this period of history. Reliance on healing teas was commonplace, but not all herbal suppliers were like the Shakers. Some suppliers were dishonest and not all physicians were regarded kindly. In a book of advice written for farmers, one grumbler said:

> Nature hath appointed remedies in a readiness for all diseases, but the craft and imbecility of man for gain surrounds us with deuced apothecary shops in which a man's life is to be sold or bought where for a little spoil they fetch their medicines from Jerusalem and out of Turkey, while, in the meantime, every poor man hath the right remedies growing in his garden: for, if men should make gardens their physicians, the physician's craft would soon decay.

Well, not quite, of course. Medical miracles are performed every day. Still, there is more than a grain of truth in what that disgruntled gentleman had to say. Those disgruntled with physicians sometimes opt for alternatives; macrobiotics is one such alternative system.

THE MACROBIOTIC WAY

It was Hippocrates (460–370 B.C.), known as the "Father of Medicine," who was the first to use the term macrobiotics. In Greek, macro means "large" or "great," and bios means life. Thus, macrobiotics signifies "great life." It was the late eighteenth century when a German physician named Christophe W. Hufeland wrote a book entitled, *Macrobiotics, or The Art of Prolonging Life*. Chances are, you've never read Hufeland's book, but you've probably heard about macrobiotics.

The macrobiotic lifestyle as we know it today is based on the findings of Sagen Ishizuka, M.D., and Yukikazu Sakurazawa. These two Japanese educators cured themselves of serious illnesses with a simple diet of brown rice, miso soup, sea vegetables, special non-traditional teas, and other wholesome foods. When

Sakurazawa came to Paris in the late 1920s, macrobiotics crept into Western consciousness. Sakurazawa changed his name to George Ohsawa and began teaching the macrobiotic lifestyle.

In 1949, Michio Kushi introduced macrobiotics to the United States. Author of many books on macrobiotics and founder of the Kushi Institute and East-West Foundation, which publishes the *East-West Journal*, Michio Kushi is an acknowledged expert on the macrobiotic lifestyle. As in all great healing traditions, the macrobiotic system mandates a healthy lifestyle designed to prevent illness and disease from developing in the first place.

The cornerstone of macrobiotics is a body-friendly diet based primarily on whole grains and vegetables, a diet that takes into consideration the inner workings of the human body. The macrobiotic diet includes bancha tea (brewed from the twigs of *Camellia sinensis*, the green tea plant), kombu tea (brewed from a sea vegetable), umeboshi tea (from pickled Japanese plums) and the more familiar dandelion root, roasted barley, and rice teas. Mu tea is another item on the macrobiotic menu. It is a blend of mild non-stimulating herbs, and is used for relieving fatigue. All traditional macrobiotic teas qualify as healing teas. Bancha tea is an especially fine preventive medicine in its own right. (For information on purchasing these teas, see Chapter 4; to obtain more information on the macrobiotic lifestyle, see page 228.)

FROM HERBAL SCIENCE TO MEDICAL SCIENCE

Today, orthodox medicine looks askance at healing teas, yet it should not. Medical science owes a lot to the plants of the fields. Approximately 70 percent of today's drugs are derived from natural substances, many of which have been used for millennia in the ancient healing systems.

For example, the drug digitoxin, used as a heart stimulant, comes from the common foxglove (*Digitalis purpurea*). As mentioned earlier, the Chinese have used it for 4,000 years. Digitoxin, the manmade pharmaceutical, is toxic, as its name proclaims, and has unwanted side effects. It must be used medically with great care. On the other hand, foxglove tea has been used against heart disease for thousands of years. Another case in point is quinine, derived from cinchona bark. It is used chiefly in the treatment of malaria. For more than 300 years, chinchona bark was the only effective remedy for malaria. It was not until 1944 that anti-malarial drugs (quinine) were first synthesized in a laboratory. However, some strains of malaria developed a resistance to the synthetics. In the 1960s, natural quinine was reinstated as the treatment of choice in certain cases.

The opium poppy (*Papaver somniferum*) offers important pain-relieving analgesics and narcotics, including morphine, codeine and thebaine, plus muscle-relaxers and that age-old treatment for diarrhea, paregoric. Laudanum, a tincture of opium, was a favorite remedy in Victorian days. No medical doctor was without a supply of this early tranquilizer. Even today, morphine, the most potent alkaloid of opium, remains the standard against which all new synthetic pain-relievers are measured.

Most recently, a new drug, taxol, derived from the Pacific yew tree has been showing great promise against cancer. Because the extract is so difficult to obtain, scientists have been trying to synthesize the active components.

And long before aspirin existed, various parts of the willow (*Salix*) were used as an anti-inflammatory agent and for relief from pain. Years ago, scientists confirmed that the salicin derived from the willow family relieves pain, reduces inflammation, and lowers fever. The herbalists knew the stunning properties offered by the willow and have used it for ages.

Chinese healers used willow leaves, Ayurvedic physicians used the bark and the berries, and European herbalists brewed willow tea to bring down a fever. Native Americans chewed the berries and used the bark in various ways. For example, they applied dried and pounded willow bark to open wounds and to the navels of newborn infants to staunch bleeding and prevent infection.

It wasn't until 1899 that salicylic acid was synthesized as acetylsalicylic acid and aspirin, as we know it today, was born. It took even longer for aspirin, hailed as a miracle drug, to come into common usage. It was the mid-1930s before aspirin became a staple in the medicine cabinets of the nation. And it all began with a steaming cup of healing tea brewed from the bark of the common willow tree.

THAT WAS THEN, THIS IS NOW

There are over a million species of plants on this sweet Earth.

Fully two-thirds of all plant species flourish in tropical rain forests, yet entire species are disappearing at an alarming rate as civilization comes ever closer to the forests. (Fully 50 thousand plant and animals species are being lost each year!) According to a spokesperson for the Rain Forest Action Coalition, subsistence farming is the primary reason for deforestation in Africa. It's hard to fault a population intent on survival. So, the trees are cut, and the undergrowth—with perhaps many medicinal treasures—is cleared. In South and Central America, the raising of cattle (for the fast-food and prepared markets), as well as subsistence farming, hydroelectric dams, mining, oil extraction, and logging are contributing heavily to the loss of the rain forests. In Asia, the rain forests are falling primarily due to logging interests.

Dedicated people are working frantically to save specimens of threatened plants from the rapidly disappearing rain forests. They hope that some new life-giving medicinals will be discovered before many plants are lost forever. The National Cancer Institute reports that 70 percent of the plants identified as useful in the treatment of cancer are found only in rain forests. Even the American Cancer Society, never before known as an organization that espouses natural medicinals, is running an on-going effort to collect plants in Belize. In this tiny Central American country, scientists are actively seeking the cooperation of the local shamans, or "wise ones," and the practicing herbalists. Their knowledge is traditionally passed from master to apprentice. If the "wise ones" who can identify the medicinal plants and prepare the compounds depart this world before their expertise can be recorded, much may be forever lost.

Spare a thought for those who are working worldwide to salvage both special species of plants and the old wisdom. With the Biblical command ringing in our ears, ". . . and the leaf thereof for medicine (Ezekiel 47:12)," it's hard not to dwell on what the world may be losing forever. Fortunately, we still have a wide variety of highly effective natural medicinals available to us, including many that have survived since ancient times. In the next chapter, Healing Teas Today, I'll spell out exactly what healing teas are, what they can do for you, and how to prepare them.

3

Healing Teas Today

As you have seen, herbs and other natural medicinals are the cornerstone of all the ancient healing traditions. They are still used worldwide today—by Chinese medical doctors, Ayurvedic vaidyas, macrobiotic practitioners, Native American healers, the shamans of South America, and in millions of households from Alaska to Zanzibar—for just one reason. They work.

A growing number of people strongly believe that Mother (Nature) knows best. Without question, the natural medicinals have some very real advantages when compared with manmade drugs. Nature's medicinals can do just about anything manmade pharmaceuticals can do, and, with very few exceptions, herbal brews and other natural medicinals are free of the adverse effects characteristic of manmade drugs. The ingredients found in nature's pharmacy are time-tested and body-friendly.

THE ADVANTAGES OF USING WHOLE HERBS

A century ago, science discovered how to isolate, identify, and extract the active elements in the herbal remedies that had been in use for thousands of years. Delighted with this new "toy," researchers convinced themselves that only one element was the source of a plant's power to heal. They proceeded to "throw the baby out with the bath water" by agreeing among themselves that the rest of the plant's constituents had to be just so many useless and inactive elements. That error was set in stone when the medical detectives then decided it would be much better to pull out the one compound they had labeled "active" and use it in their research against disease, rather than continue investigating the ways in which the whole plant worked.

Better? No. Easier? Yes. That's how the pharmaceutical companies grew into the powerful force they have become. Yet, even in this day and age, with the heavy reliance Western medicine has on engineered and synthetic medicines, more than 25 percent of all prescription drugs in the United States are derived from herbs and plants.

While many life-saving drugs have been discovered, the vast majority of commonly used medications come with many potentially dangerous side effects. Many of these synthesized drugs emphasize a quick fix without looking at the long-term effects. By isolating a single active ingredient, researchers ignore the delicate balance nature has developed in these plants over millions of years. It turns out that a lot of the best stuff may, in fact, go into the trash barrel. Today, we know the whole herb contains necessary companion-compounds that help the so-called "active" element work better while, at the same time, soften its sometimes harsh effects. The "working" parts of the plant—whether roots, flowers, buds, leaves, or bark—are the repository of more than just one active compound, as well as a variety of still more elements that act as potentiators and buffers.

Andrew Weil, M.D., has had much experience comparing the effectiveness of the whole plant with a pharmaceutical extract taken from the same plant. In his book *Health and Healing*, Dr. Weil says, "Whenever I have had a chance to experience treatment with a plant and treatment with a refined derivative of the plant, I have found the latter [the refined derivative] to be more dangerous and sometimes less useful."

This is not to suggest that the world would be better off without pharmaceutical drugs. There will always be times when only a quick-acting broad-spectrum drug—whether plant-based or engineered from scratch in the lab—will do the job. If your condition is serious enough to warrant attention by a physician, chances are you'll be quick to welcome prescription drugs.

On the other hand, there will always be times when a safe and gentle healing tea is the nicer choice. It's up to you to weigh the benefits of each approach and determine when the time is right for sipping a steaming cup of natural medicinal brew.

For example, if you suffer from insomnia and you're sick of being awake while the rest of the world is off to dreamland, you're liable to resort to almost anything to get a good night's sleep. Tossing and turning is no fun. The desperate need for rest may send you out into the dark searching for a twenty-four-hour drugstore where you can find an over-the-counter sleep aid.

Arriving home, you pop a couple of pills and settle down with a sigh of relief. This stuff may zonk you out, but you might as well hit yourself in the head with a hammer. You'll have the same type of headache in the morning. Because of the concentrated chemicals in these preparations, you'll probably awaken with a drug-induced hangover and feel groggy, dragged out, and miserable all day.

Even worse, some sleep-inducers are so strong that you sleep without dreaming. Without experiencing the fourth-stage deep REM sleep of dreams, the human body reacts with nervous irritability. If you fail to achieve REM sleep for too many nights, tremors develop. Then, too, you may develop dependency on sleep aids that will force you to choose between sleepless nights or more chemical-induced nightmarish symptoms.

There is a better way. Several herbal teas come to mind. Chamomile, for example, was used by the ancient Egyptians for its relaxing effects. By the 1600s, chamomile was in wide use in Europe, and it's still much appreciated today around the world. A cup of chamomile tea soothes the restless spirit and helps the body ease into the natural state of relaxation that fosters sleep.

St. John's wort is another herb that has been in use for centuries. As every insomniac knows, it's hard to go to sleep if you're anxious about falling asleep in the first place. St. John's wort is traditionally used to relieve anxiety and lift the spirits, as well as to treat insomnia. Even more reassuring is the fact that studies have shown this root to improve the quality of sleep.

Of all the herbs, valerian is the champion sedative of historic fame. Recent findings have substantiated the old wisdom. Valerian not only relieves insomnia, it improves the quality of sleep, cuts down the number of times an insomniac awakens in the night, and doesn't leave the user with a nervous headache in the morning. (Incidentally, if you have trouble falling asleep, don't bother making notes. You'll find more on all three of these herbs in Chapter 6, A Selection of Natural Medicinals.)

You can even be a teetotaler *and* get the reputed benefits of red wine. Andrew Waterhouse, Ph.D., of the University of California at Davis has analyzed the biologically active components of various beverages. He has found that tea has about the same amount of catechins as red wine; catechins are antioxidants that seem to help prevent the clogging of arteries by reducing the negative effects of LDL cholesterol.

If you must select between a manmade conglomeration of chemicals with some really nasty side effects or one of Mother Nature's nicely formulated remedies, the better way is obvious, isn't it?

ATTITUDES ARE CHANGING

There's a wide and growing sense of dissatisfaction with how allopathic (orthodox) medicine handles many of our health-care needs. In the not-too-distant past, the patient looked on the doctor as all-knowing, and his advice was never questioned. But the doctor isn't a "god" anymore. We're not only asking questions, we're not happy with the answers we're getting. And, more often than not, the too-busy medical professional can't take the time to really address all our concerns.

Certainly, we do not plan to turn up our noses at the technological advances we've gained in the past fifty years. The latest in surgical techniques and the quite amazing diagnostic tools that have been developed are stunning achievements, available for our benefit should the need arise.

It's the reliance of orthodox medicine on prescription drugs with their dangerous and even harmful side effects that's turning a lot of people off. That's why more and more people are investigating the old ways and practicing some very effective self-care health-care, including sipping a cup of healing tea instead of taking a manmade drug.

HOW HEALING TEAS WORK

Natural medicinals can cause a favorable alteration of body chemistry, bring the internal systems back into balance, and support the body while they hasten healing. Nature's medicines can cleanse and detoxify, alleviate pain, reduce fever, induce sweating, boost the defensive forces of the body, fight infection, sweeten a sour stomach, calm a disturbed intestinal tract, expel worms, cure scurvy, fight cancer, ease involuntary spasms, stem hemorrhage both internally and externally, strengthen and stabilize a faulty heart, increase the discharge of urine, cause vomiting, induce coughing to bring up phlegm, dissolve blockages, support a tired liver, calm the nerves, help with a difficult childbirth, even put you to sleep or wake you up.

Healing teas have specific medicinal properties, depending on their ingredients. Pharmaceutical drugs, whether over-the-counter or prescription, have specific medicinal properties, depending on their ingredients. Remember, the herbalist is the forerunner of the pharmacist. That's why, very often, the man-made "cousin" mimics the effects of the natural medicinals, not the other way around. The terminology is different because the old ways still prevail in the world of healing teas.

Healing teas are not drugs. Although top-quality natural medicinals have the ability to address both the symptoms and root cause of a health problem, they do not enter the body and go charging around, zapping germs, and jolting internal systems into hyperactive changes. Don't expect quick-fix symptomatic-relief.

The majority of natural medicinals work over a period of time. Herbal ingredients support the body in natural ways by bolstering the body's most basic internal systems. These herbal substances allow the body's natural defense mechanisms to gain control and clear away the cause of the problem. And, in many cases, they provide safe and effective relief from annoying symptoms. Although it may seem as if it's taking a very long time to achieve results when you start taking healing teas, the slower process allows the body to adjust at a more natural speed.

Herbal support in the form of healing teas can make a difference in how you feel in three to six days. Monitor your reactions. Gains come in such tiny increments that you may not be aware you're feeling better unless you're looking for change.

If you are trying healing teas for a chronic or long-standing problem, natural medicinals can be of great benefit, but they will take time to work. Master herbalists say herbs require one month of healing-time for every year you've been wrestling with a problem.

PREPARING HEALING TEAS

There are many ways to use nature's medicinals. No matter what method is employed, the idea is to release, extract, and activate all the useful properties of the plant. For the most part, that's accomplished with liquid. In other words, even poultices, plasters, and ointments start as teas.

A word of caution. Never use tap water. There are just too many chemicals in tap water that can interact with and alter the working properties of healing teas. Always use bottled water when preparing home remedies.

When preparing healing teas, the same rules apply as laid out in Chapter 1 for Traditional Sipping Teas. Don't use an aluminum kettle, and don't steep teas in plastic or any metal other than stainless steel. For a fresh taste without taint, use china, glass, or crockery.

You'll need a larger quantity of plant parts when using fresh herbs. This makes sense when you remember that the properties of dried plant parts are concentrated. Powdered herbs are even more concentrated. To learn how much of an herb you need for various applications, be guided by the instructions on the box or, in the case of loose herbs sold by the ounce, by the on-duty herbalist at the shop where you are making the purchase.

In Chapter 6, A Selection of Natural Medicinals, you'll find a comprehensive listing of medicinal herbs that brew into healing teas. If you brew up a cup and find you don't care for the taste of a particular herb, it will help to remember that the purpose of a healing tea is to support your body in positive ways. Many medicinal herbs are bland and taste vaguely of earthy fields and grassy meadows. Some herbs are faintly sweet and smooth, but others are bitter on the tongue. When you add anything to a healing tea, be aware that the addition will interact chemically and change the properties of the brew. Even honey will affect the working quality of the tea, but if you simply must add something, make it a drizzle of honey.

A Word About Measuring

If you read a variety of herbals, you'll find that directions for measuring herbs are sometimes given in ounces, sometimes in grams, and sometimes in teaspoons. There's a reason for this. Since way back when, the scientific community has used the metric system of measuring, in which a gram is the primary unit of weight. American cooks are much more likely to measure in teaspoons or ounces. The situation becomes complicated when you consider that the term "ounce" is used for both dry and liquid measure.

You can use your kitchen measuring cup to measure the eight ounces of freshly boiled water required to brew a single cup of healing tea. However, because the standard measuring cup is designed to measure liquids, you can't use the same measuring cup to measure, say, one ounce of a particular herb. In other words, you can't arrive at the precise measurement of a dry substance by using a measuring cup designed to measure liquid.

There's another factor to consider when measuring herbs: the way an herb has been dried and processed. For example, some loose herbs are crushed and powdery. Some natural medicinals are crumbled, but retain some shape. Your kitchen measuring spoons will be fine for measuring the specified amounts of these herbs. But some plant parts are crudely cut into bits and pieces of varying sizes, and some—primarily the root herbs—are cut into chunks or very large pieces. Spoons just won't "cut it."

No matter what form a natural medicinal takes, the best way to arrive at the precise measurement of dry herb is to weigh it. That's not as intimidating as it may sound.

You can find kitchen scales in just about any mall. Such scales are available in three basic types:

1. ***Spring action.*** *These are usually the least expensive scales, ranging in price from $5 to $25. Over time, however, the springs tend to stretch, and the readings may become inaccurate.*

2. ***Old-fashioned weights and balance.*** *This classic measuring device used by apothecaries and pharmacists for generations*

works by balancing an item placed on one platform with a fixed weight on the other. Traditionally, the weights are made of brass. While these scales can be attractive in a kitchen setting, they may be a little pricey. You can pay anwhere from $50 upwards.

3. **Digital.** *Technological advances have brought us scales with digital readouts—place an item on the platform and the weight appears as if by magic. These scales cost from $50 to $100.*

Scales can be purchased in kitchenware sections of depart-ment stores, shops specializing in kitchen gadgets, gourmet shops, and antique stores. I suggest that you start with the cheapest scale. If you are seriously considering becoming an expert at brewing healing teas, the small investment is worth it. If you then find you're using the scale often, consider investing in one that's top-of-the-line.

If, however, you believe that tea is to be brewed using a teaspoon, this book provides teaspoon measurements as well as ounce and gram measurements for every natural medicinal dis-cussed in Part II.

Please do use a measuring spoon; teaspoons that come with flatware are too variable in size. You can purchase measuring spoons wherever cookware is sold. Be sure the set you buy has tablespoon, half-tablespoon, teaspoon, half-teaspoon, quarter-tea-spoon, and eighth-teaspoon measures. Some sets even have a spoon that measures a pinch, which is less than one-eighth tea-spoon. Measuring spoons are available in metal or plastic; I recom-mend you get a metal set.

When measuring herbs with spoons, be aware that directions may specify level, rounded, or heaping spoonfuls. When the con-tents are level with the top edge of the spoon, you have a level teaspoon. In a rounded teaspoon, the contents form a slight mound in the middle. When the contents form a significant mound, you have a heaping teaspoon.

As you gain experience measuring herbs, you should find that your confidence in preparing tea increases. Should you ever have any questions about measurement, you might contact a profes-sional herbalist or staff members in an herb shop.

The following are general instructions covering the most common methods of using natural pharmaceuticals:

Bath

The methods of preparing a full bath, a sitz bath, or a wash are the same. Only the proportions differ.

For a full bath, soak approximately 7 ounces of dried herbs or 6 quarts of fresh herb parts overnight in enough cold water to cover the herbs. In the morning, heat the mixture and strain off the liquid. Add the infusion to a full bath and enjoy a 20-minute soak. Upon leaving the bath, don't bother to dry off. Go to bed and cover up warmly to induce perspiration. Relax for an hour. If you doze off, so much the better.

For a sitz bath, you'll need about 3 ounces of dried herbs, or 2 1/2 quarts of fresh herb parts. Soak, warm, and strain as above. It might seem terribly obvious to tell you that you sit in a sitz bath. The level of water should cover the area of the kidneys.

For a wash, use about 1 ounce of dried herbs, or 2 cups of fresh herb parts. Soak, warm, and strain as above.

Infused waters prepared for a sitz bath or wash may be rewarmed and used three times in all before they lose their potency.

Decoction

A decoction is needed to release the deeper essences from hard or coarse substances, such as barks, roots, stems, and twigs. Steeping and leaching won't do it, but simmering will.

The procedure for making a decoction is depicted in Figure 3.1. Begin by putting the raw materials into a pot (stainless steel or enamel is preferred) and add fresh water. Simmer uncovered until the water content is reduced by $\frac{1}{3}$, usually about 10 to 20 minutes. Because these broad instructions will vary depending on the density of the basic ingredients, please be guided by the information printed on the box or by the shopkeeper as to how much raw material and how much water to use. Strain before drinking.

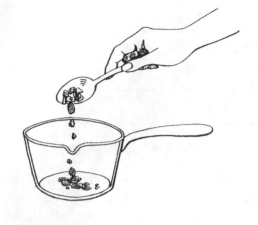

1. Place raw materials
   into a pot and add
   fresh water.

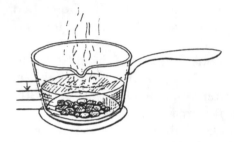

2. Simmer uncovered
   until water content
   reduces by one
   third.

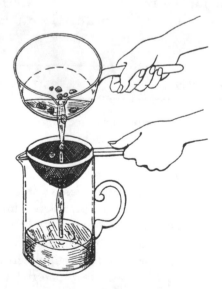

3. Place strainer over
   a glass pitcher.
   Pour decoction
   through the
   strainer into the
   pitcher.

Figure 3.1   Decoction Procedure

Fomentation

A fomentation may be used to treat swellings, pain, colds, and flu. Soak a soft white towel or cloth in the desired hot tea (infusion). Leave the towel wet but not dripping. Apply the fomentation as hot as the patient can tolerate. To hold in the heat, cover the tea-soaked towel with a warm piece of flannel, or even another towel. Repeat and reapply as needed.

Infusion

An infusion is just another name for tea. When you put a teabag in a cup and add hot water, you're making an infusion. This is the easiest and most common way of preparing a healing tea. If you are using loose herbs, the general rule of thumb is to use one heaping teaspoon of active dried ingredients (leaves, blossoms, flowers) to one cup of water. (In Part II, measurements for tea preparation are given in teaspoons; ounces and grams appear in parentheses.)

Pour freshly boiled water over the herb parts (a heaping teaspoon of dried ingredients to 8 ounces of water). Cover and steep for three to five minutes. Strain. If you will be taking a steeped infusion thoughout the day, prepare the entire quantity at one time and put it in a thermos to keep the tea at a comfortable sipping temperature. Rinse the thermos first with hot water so you don't cool the tea by putting it into a cold container.

Infusion, Cold

Some ingredients lose medicinal properties when heat is applied, but you can make a tea nonetheless. To prepare a cold infusion, measure the recommended quantity of ingredients and soak overnight in cold water. The following morning, you may warm slightly to sipping temperature, if you wish. Strain before using.

Infusion, Hot and Cold

On occasion, you'll find a plant that contains some elements that are released by heat, and some that are leached out by soaking in cold water overnight. Here's how to get around that dilemma.

First, soak the recommended amount of herb in just half the amount of cold water specified for preparing tea. The following morning, strain off and keep the liquid and retain the residue separately. Now bring half the recommended amount of water to a boil and pour over the leached herbs. Allow the mixture to steep, covered, for 3 minutes. Strain and combine the hot infusion with the cold in a tempered glass container. (Figure 3.2 depicts the procedure.) In this way, the active elements released by both heat and cold are extracted.

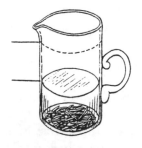

1. In a tempered glass pitcher, soak recommended amount of herb in half the amount of water normally specified. Let soak overnight.

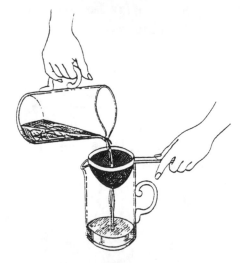

2. The following morning, strain off the liquid by pouring mixture through a strainer into a second tempered glass pitcher. Retain both the liquid and the herbal residue separately.

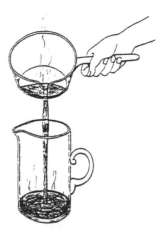

3. Place the herbal residue
   back in the first pitcher.
   Then, measure out the
   same amount of fresh
   water used in step 1, and
   bring to a boil. Pour the
   boiling water into the first
   pitcher, over the herbal
   residue.

4. Cover the pitcher and allow
   the mixture to steep for
   3 minutes.

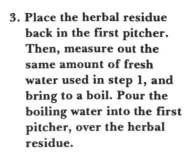

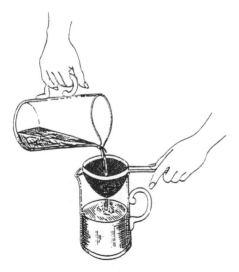

5. Place a strainer over the
   second pitcher, which
   contains the cold infusion
   from step 2. Pour the hot
   herbal mixture from the
   first pitcher through the
   strainer to combine the
   two infusions. The herbal
   residue can be discarded.

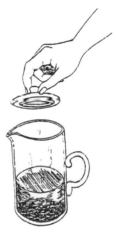

Figure 3.2   Hot and Cold Infusion Procedure

Juice

Yes, you can juice herbs. The fresh juices are wonderfully potent. The resulting drops can be diluted in herbal teas, sipping teas, or water for internal use and, depending on the plant, the juice can help clear certain skin conditions when used externally.

To juice natural medicinals, wash a suitable quantity of plant parts under cold, running water. Place them, still wet, in a juice extractor. If necessary, scissor the pieces into a uniform size.

Juices should be used immediately after they are extracted. However, you can put the liquid into a tightly sealed bottle and hold refrigerated for several days without an appreciable loss of properties.

Oil

Making an herbal oil is easy. Place flowers or herb parts loosely in a glass (not plastic) bottle. Slowly add cold-pressed virgin olive oil until the oil level is an inch above the herbs or flower heads. Cork tightly.

Allow the bottle to stand in a very warm place (80°F or warmer) for 2 weeks. Put it near the stove to gather warmth from cooking, or give it a sunbath on hot days. Just remember to bring it in before evening cools the air. Upend the bottle and turn it end-to-end daily.

The quality of the blend depends on the quality of the oil you use. Please use virgin olive oil only. Don't substitute common vegetable cooking or salad oils. Hydrogenated and partially hydrogenated oils and processed foods containing this type of fat have no place in my house. It would take an entire book to tell you everything that's wrong with the chemically processed dietary oils and fats that line the shelves of the supermarkets in this country. For one thing, all the essential fatty acids (EFAs) the body needs daily (and can't manufacture) have been processed out. However, as they say, that's another story.

Ointment

Not so very long ago, there wasn't a drugstore on every corner. Every housewife not only knew how to make soap, she knew how to make pain-relieving ointments and soothing salves.

To prepare an ointment, heat 2 cups of pure lard (not vegetable shortening) to french-frying temperature, around 385 to 395°F. Add 4 big handfuls of finely crumbled dry herbs or 6 handfuls of chopped fresh herb parts (scissors make it easy to chop them) to the hot fat. The herbs will crackle and sizzle and splatter, so beware of spitting fat. Stir to blend. After 1 minute, remove from heat and cover. Allow the mixture to rest overnight.

Next morning, heat gently to liquify and stir in 4 tablespoons of virgin olive oil. The olive oil will help prevent the ointment from solidifying into a rock-hard mass. Squeeze through a cheesecloth to remove the residue. Place the filtered ointment in crockery or glass (not plastic) containers and allow to harden.

Plaster

If you think of grandmother's famous mustard plaster, you'll see why a plaster is a "sandwich." Plasters are typically made with strong rubefacient materials that have the potential to redden and irritate the skin.

Prepare the herb parts as for either a steamed or pulped poultice, but place the warm mass of pulverized herbs between two layers of cloth before applying to the desired area. Depending on the herbs used, plasters can be left in place for an extended period of time, even overnight.

Poultice, Pulped

The procedure for preparing a pulped poultice is depicted in Figure 3.3. Place a quantity of fresh plant material on a clean white cloth. Fold so plant material is inside. Crush with a rolling pin (or heavy bottle). Crushing the herbs directly onto the cloth retains

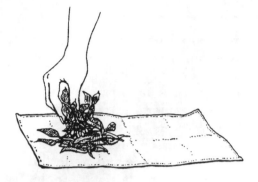

1. **Place the plant material on one half of a clean, white, rectangular cloth.**

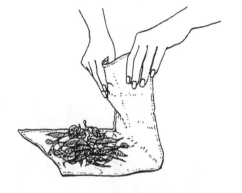

2. **Fold the cloth in half to cover the plant material.**

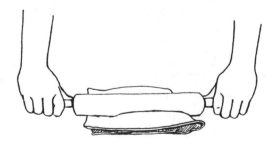

3. **Roll a rolling pin over the folded cloth to crush the plant material.**

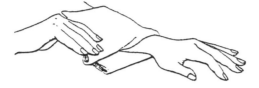

4. **Apply the poultice to the affected area. (In this case the affected area is the forearm.)**

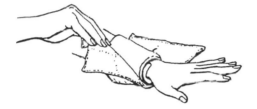

5. **Wrap the poultice with a second cloth or bandage to hold in body heat and keep in place.**

Figure 3.3   Making a Pulped Poultice

all the juices, thus improving the efficiency of the poultice. Apply the poultice to the affected area and overwrap with a cover to hold in body heat. A pulped poultice can stay in place overnight.

Poultice, Steamed

The procedure for preparing a steamed poultice is depicted in Figure 3.4. To prepare a poultice with fresh herbs, place a colander over a pot of rapidly boiling water. Make sure that the water will not touch the material to be placed in the colander.

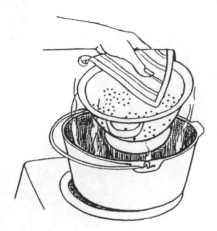

1. Place colander over a pot of
   boiling water. Make sure that
   the water will not touch the
   material to be placed in the
   colander.

2. Layer the herb parts in the
   colander, and reduce heat to
   simmer.

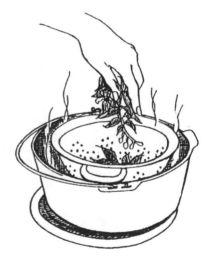

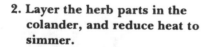

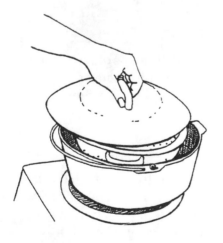

3. While water is simmering, cover
   the pot and colander to keep the
   steam in. The steam will wilt and
   soften the plant parts.

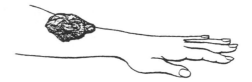

4. **Remove the softened herbal mixture from the colander and wait at least 10 minutes for the mass to cool somewhat before applying. Carefully place the warm mixture onto the affected area.**

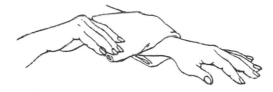

5. **Wrap a clean folded cloth around the affected area to hold in heat and keep the mixture in place.**

Figure 3.4 Making a Steamed Poultice

Layer the herb parts in the colander, reduce the heat to simmering temperature, cover, and allow the steam to wilt and penetrate the plant parts. About 10 minutes after removing from heat, apply the warmed herbal mass to the affected area. Cover to hold in the heat. When the poultice cools, reapply as needed.

Salve

Blend together 3 ounces of finely pulverized herb parts (Grand-mother used a mortar and pestle), 7 ounces of cocoa butter (or lard), and 1 ounce of beeswax. When nicely blended, simmer over very low heat in a covered pot for 1 to 2 hours. Remove from heat. As the mixture cools, it will firm up. If you find the end result is too soft, next time add another half-ounce of beeswax.

Tincture

Tinctures employ alcohol to extract the active properties of a natural medicinal. It's easy to make a tincture at home. Loosely fill a glass (not plastic) bottle with fresh or dried herbs. Add pure food-grade spirits (not rubbing alcohol); vodka is best. Cork the bottle and allow it to stand in a warm place (around 70°F) for at least 2 weeks. Give the bottle a shake every day. After 2 weeks have passed, the tincture is ready for use. Tinctures are often given as drops in tea or taken diluted in a little water. They may also be useful in a compress or when a cooling massage is needed.

If you see a bottled medicinal that says "tincture," you can be sure it's alcohol-based. Many herbal extracts on the market are actually tinctures. Check the label if you want to avoid alcohol.

IN CONCLUSION

Now that you know what healing teas can do and the many ways there are to use the natural medicinals, let's go shopping. In the next chapter, I'll tell you what to look for in raw ingredients and what to watch out for.

4

Shopping for Healing Teas

As you have seen in earlier chapters, healing teas have been used with great benefit for millennia. Without the experiences passed down by the master physicians of ages past who both compounded and brewed their own medicinal teas, our knowledge of healing plants would be meager indeed.

Please keep in mind that the physicians of antiquity formulated their healing teas with great care. They were very particular about the apothecary shop they patronized, too. To ensure that the healing brews the doctors personally compounded and dispensed to their patients were biologically active, the healers of old insisted on herbs that were organically pure, recently dried, and fully potent. That's what you must do, too.

Long ago, in a warning against "false drugs," the Chinese scholar P'ei-lan set down this warning: "Sellers of drugs have two eyes; Prescribers of drugs have one eye; Takers of drugs have no eyes." This seems to be the Chinese equivalent of the old expression, "Let the buyer beware."

INGREDIENT SHOPPING

Before you go shopping for the herbal ingredients you need to brew your own teas, there are several points to keep in mind. Remember, the herbs you need to brew healing teas are not subject to the same regulations that govern lab-produced drugs. There's no "watchdog" committee making sure an ounce of natural ingredients will always contain a standardized amount of pure and potent biologically active elements. If the herbs are old, they are less likely to be active. Irradiated herbs may also not be "up to snuff." There is some evidence that irradiating foods can affect essential fatty acids, amino acids, and vitamins. To find out if the herbs have been irradiated, check for a symbol of a circle whose circumferance is composed of five fat lines and which contains a stylized flower. If you are new to healing teas and herbal medicines, take some time to explore various sources of raw materials. Fresh-picked herbs are sometimes hard to find, but their use is one way to ensure that all the properties you want are present in the plant and are fully active. Herb shops or herbalists can offer one-stop shopping. Check the Yellow Pages of your telephone directory under such headings as Herbs, Herbalists, Botanicals.

You can also browse the Yellow Pages for some organic farmers in your area that specialize in herbs. For the most part, organic farms are family owned and operated. The farmers will welcome your call. If your first call reaches someone who isn't cultivating herbs, chances are that person can refer you to a local farmer who does specialize in the natural medicinals.

You might also check out small markets that feature fresh produce and ask what medicinal herbs they carry. Here again, expect a friendly welcome over the phone. If you've hit the wrong market, ask for a referral. You'll probably get one. Markets specializing in products from Asia are excellent sources of fresh herbs.

If you are unsuccessful in finding a source of garden-fresh herbs, not to worry. Dried herbs are three times as powerful as fresh herb parts. For centuries, healing teas have been brewed with dried herbs.

Be aware that even dried herb parts are subject to deterioration. Some herbs are sensitive to light and are best stored in tightly sealed tins, not glass. All herbs lose their original potency very quickly on exposure to air. For full activity, dried herb parts should be no older than six or eight months.

A dusty out-of-the-way herb shop displaying a wide array of

herbs may be perfectly charming and appear "old world," but it probably won't be a good source for active herbs. If the proprietor sells only a few ounces of one herb or another every few weeks, chances are his stock is old and less active than it should be. One way to tell if dried herbs are too old to brew into an effective healing tea is to apply the "sniff test." Herbs that are recently dried won't smell strong, but they should still retain a whiff of their original scent. If they have no aroma at all or smell like a room that's been closed up too long, there's a possibility they have "expired."

Dried herb parts for brewing teas aren't the only way the natural medicinals are marketed. You'll also find herbals in extract or tincture form, usually in a bottle with an eye-dropper in the lid. It's easy enough to squeeze a few drops in a cup of tea, but think twice about these offerings. The extraction process is sometimes accomplished with the aid of chemical solvents. Read the label to find out what extractant was used. Tinctures employ alcohol to leach certain elements from the whole herb. If you want to avoid alcohol, avoid tinctures. I favor the more traditional approach to brewing healing teas. Fresh herbs, dried herbs of recent origin, and/or dried and powdered herbs will always be of much greater benefit than extracts or tinctures.

To make sure of the highest degree of purity and potency in your herbal ingredients, visit one of the larger herb shops or health-food stores in your area. Pick one with a lot of traffic and a knowledgeable staff, then be guided by staff members' expertise.

Here's one more word to the wise: Don't congratulate yourself on searching out the lowest-priced herbal ingredients to brew your healing teas. This is one instance where quality and care in processing show up in price. Expect to pay a little more for the best. And don't begrudge it. If you want your teas to be of full benefit, spend for quality ingredients.

It is not the purpose of this book to recommend any particular brand of herbs for brewing healing teas, so you need to do a little homework. If you don't find any local shops that seem to suit your needs, you might want to take a look at a book entitled *The Herb Companion: Wishbook and Resource Guide* by Bobbi A. McRae. This book will refer you to the sources for any herbs you may be seeking for brewing healing teas, plus a whole lot more. The book also lists sources of plants and seeds for growing your own "fixings" for medicinal brews. If this book isn't readily available in your area, see page 227 for an address and phone number so you can order it by mail.

SHOPPING FOR READY-MADE HEALING TEAS

One of the difficulties of blending your own healing teas is the problem of arriving at the perfect amount of active ingredients per cupful. As I explained earlier, loose herbs will always contain varying quantities of active elements, depending on how they were grown, how they were processed, how they were stored, and how old they are when you buy them.

You can sidestep those pitfalls by purchasing healing teas that are scientifically blended and continually tested to make sure that each cup of steeped tea delivers the optimum amount of active constituents. Here's my vote for the best of the ready-mades: I highly recommend the line of teas offered by the Traditional Medicinals Herb Tea Company. This company not only offers an excellent selection of blended medicinal teas, it has also gone to the trouble and expense of having its Smooth Move Tea approved by the United States Food and Drug Administration (FDA) as an over-the-counter drug product. Traditional Medicinals offers a number of other preblended teas including Breathe Easy, Cold Care P.M., PMS Tea, and a variety of teas that fall under the following headings: Beverage Tea Blends, Gourmet Herbal Teas, and Traditional Classic Teas. These other teas are not FDA-approved medicinals and do not carry health advice. This means that the company can't tell you the good things they can do for your body, but I can. That's why I want to single out two teas for honorable mention. They qualify as healing teas in their own right.

Golden Green Tea. Green tea (*Camellia sinensis*) has wonderfully healthy properties. (See page 150 for more information.) This delightful blend contains both green tea and lemon grass.

Pau d'Arco. This South American bark remedy has been in use for centuries. Recent scientific findings validating the ancient wisdom show this is indeed a remedy of heroic proportions. (See page 178 for more information.)

You'll find Traditional Medicinal healing teas in health-food stores, organic produce markets, and even in a few enlightened supermarkets. If you don't care to shop for the raw ingredients with which to blend your own healing teas, it will be worth your while to make a few phone calls to find a local source of Traditional Medicinals. If all else fails, you'll find the address and phone number of this firm on page 226. The company will be happy to send you a list of stores in your area that carry its products.

Crystal Star Herbal Nutrition is another fine company with a line of preblended medicinal herbal teas. Crystal Star is as fussy as I am about the ingredients put into its healing teas. The company uses organically grown herbs or those found in the wild as much as possible, augmented with fresh-dried locally grown herbs, plus some historically valuable imported Chinese herbs. Crystal Star prides itself on frequent purchases of small amounts of herbs, rather than bulk purchases that would save money at the expense of quality. If you're interested in knowing more about the company's healing teas and other herbal formulas, see page 225 for the address and phone number.

The Seelect Herb Tea Company also offers a selection of healing teas. The company packages loose herbal teas and has a selection of many medicinal herbs in tea bags as well, but each herb stands alone. Seelect does not offer preblended herbal formulas. See page 225 for the address and phone number.

Under the heading "The Macrobiotic Way," in Chapter 2, I brought the healing teas of Japan to your attention. The fixings for these medicinal brews can be found in most major health-food stores. However, if you run into problems locating a source, markets that cater to an Asian clientele will have these very popular and very healthy teas. For more information on the macrobiotic approach to health, including the healing teas of Japan, see page 228. You'll find the addresses and phone numbers of two organizations that will be happy to direct you to trained teachers and counselors in your area.

Also in Chapter 2, I told you about the ancient Ayurvedic system of healing that has been used in India since time immemorial. I don't know of any source for the Indian herbs necessary to blend your own teas. However, you're not out of luck. If you are interested in sampling some ancient Ayurvedic traditional teas prepared according to 4,000-year-old instructions, there are some ready-made teas on the market. The names of the following three mind-body balancing teas of India are registered trademarks of Maharishi Ayur-Ved Teas:

Kapha Tea. This stimulating tea is traditionally taken by everyone during those times of the year when the weather is cold and wet. In addition, it is particularly recommended for those with an excess of Kapha dosha, typically those who are overweight, and those who feel slow and lethargic, overweight or not.

Pitta Tea. This cooling tea is traditionally taken by all when the weather is hot. In addition, it is particularly recommended for those with an excess of Pitta dosha, typically those who are irritable and impatient, those with sensitive skin, and those who always feel hot, even when others are comfortable.

Vata Tea. This calming tea is traditionally taken when the weather is cold and dry. In addition, it is particularly recommended for those with an excess of Vata dosha, typically those who are restless or stressed when traveling. It is also recommended for those individuals who have trouble falling asleep and who seldom sleep through the night.

If you would like to know more about the teas and other herbal products of India, see page 227 for appropriate addresses and phone numbers. I'm also very pleased to tell you that the Maharishi Ayur-Ved people will send you a free mind-body evaluation form you can use to determine your dosha, plus some material that promises the secrets of restoring balance for your mind-body type. All you have to do is ask. You'll find that address and phone number on page 227, too.

For still more 4,000-year-old Ayurvedic teas, look to the Ancient Healing Ways people. They offer some interesting formulas designed to, in their words, "treat the whole person, including the five elements and seven chakras." I particularly like the company's Echinacea Fitness Tea formula. It includes echinacea, ginger, pau d'arco, and astralagus. Other specialty healing teas from this line include Male Vitality Tea, Women's Tea, and Ginseng Energy. Ancient Healing Ways has a very nice color catalog, free for the asking. See page 228 for information on contacting this company.

TERMINOLOGY

When reading the information companies send you or when out shopping, you will need to know the lingo. Tea terminology is different because the old ways still prevail in the world of healing teas. To give you an example, I'll return to aspirin, so well-known it needs no introduction. As everyone knows, aspirin is used medically to bring down a fever and reduce pain and inflammation. The bottle says aspirin is a pain reliever for the temporary relief of minor aches and pains, and so it is. Pop a couple of aspirins every few hours and a fever goes down and headache or minor body and muscle aches are relieved.

The properties of a healing tea brewed from willow bark are the same. But, in the parlance of the herbalist, willow bark tea is a febrifuge (fever-reducer) and anodyne (pain-reliever). Sip a cup of willow tea every few hours, and fever is reduced and aches and pains are relieved.

An introduction to the terms that have been used down through the ages will be useful. Let's say you're standing in a health-food store looking at boxes of loose herbs. One says it contains a carminative. The box might contain anise, caraway, cloves, dill, ginger, or mint—my personal favorite. You'll want to know that a cup of aromatic carminative tea taken after a heavy dinner aids digestion, relieves a gassy stomach, and reduces flatulence.

Most of the common terms you're likely to find when shopping for ingredients for healing teas are defined below. Some you'll never need, but they are included for their interesting historical asides. I'm intensely curious about the old ways. Perhaps you are, too. If so, enjoy.

Abortifacients. As the name suggests, abortifacients are used for brewing teas long believed capable of causing abortion. In times gone by, so-called "ladies of quality" sent their most discreet servants scurrying down the alley to the local potion-pusher to purchase abor-vitae, cotton, juniper, tansy, or pennyroyal in the hope of interrupting an unwanted pregnancy. Even in intense concentration, these brews were only occasionally successful. More often than not, the only thing that happened was that "milady" suffered terrible cramping and severe gastrointestinal distress.

Alterative. An alterative substance is a plant that works gradually to alter body chemistry. Its effect is slow and sure, but not immediately noticeable.

Anodyne. An anodyne is a pain-reliever. While the willow is mild in action, many herbs properly classified as anodynes are heavy narcotics and can be dangerous. The opium poppy is a case in point.

Anthelmintic. Anthelmintics (and vermifuges) are plant medicines that expel worms. Intestinal parasites were once a huge problem, especially in the South where people often went barefoot while working the fields and walked unpaved roads without shoes.

Antipyretic. If you are familiar with the term "pyromaniac," you can figure this one out. An antipyretic fights fever and helps prevent it from recurring when taken periodically.

Antiscorbutic. You'll probably never need an antiscorbutic to prevent or cure scurvy, but our ancestors did. Teas once used to treat scurvy include dandelion root, sarsaparilla, and vitamin-C-rich lemon.

Apierient. See Laxative.

Aromatic. As you undoubtedly know, aromatic substances have a sweet or spicy aroma and usually have a pleasant, pungent taste. Aromatics are often added to compound teas to make the "medicine go down" easier. They also stimulate digestion. It's not only their flavor that makes them desirable either. The scent of plants such as ginger, sweetflag, mint, cloves, nutmeg, and caraway provides a swift lift to flagging spirits. Aromatherapy isn't new, you know. Not so very long ago, many healers called for specific sweet-smelling flowers in a sickroom.

Astringent. Astringent herbs contract tissues and help slow down the runaway discharge of body fluids, including blood. Astringent substances are indicated in the case of hemorrhage, dysentery or diarrhea.

Native Americans powdered the root of the skunk cabbage, which they called *skota*, and applied it to a running wound to stem bleeding. I will not be discussing this herb, but you might be interested to know that skunk cabbage is poisonous if taken internally.

Blood-purifier. In days gone by, herbalists used this term when referring to an herb that removed toxins from the blood.

Carminative. I've already explained that a carminative is a stomach-sweetener and digestive aid that reduces flatulence.

Carthartic. See Laxative.

Cordial. Cordials use alcohol to leach out the active properties of a medicinal substance. Blackberry brandy, which is really a cordial, was once the remedy of choice against diarrhea. It not only tasted delicious, it worked. A "wineglassful" of cordial every day was long believed beneficial to the heart. Now science has validated this herbal prescription. Recent research shows that moderate intake of an alcoholic beverage benefits the heart by increasing the amount of HDL (high density lipoproteins), the "good" cholesterol that keeps arteries clean.

Corroborant. See Tonic.

Demulcent. These teas are soothing to irritated tissues, especially of the digestive tract. They are oily or mucilaginous in texture. Marshmallow, indeed all the members of the mallow (*Malva*) family, have been used since ancient times to soothe a sore throat, coat the stomach, and calm a disturbed intestinal tract.

Deobstruent. As the name suggests, a deobstruent tea is historically assigned the task of clearing an obstruction in the natural ducts of the body.

Depurant. A depurant helps purify various internal systems, (i.e., blood, liver, kidneys, intestinal tract, lungs), depending on the herb used. Many compound tonics employ a cleansing depurant as part of their ingredients.

Diaphoretic. A diaphoretic (or sudorific) tea stimulates copious perspiration to help rid the body of toxins. People of many nationalities—most notably the Finns, from whom we borrowed the sauna—use sweat baths to promote health.

Diuretic. Diuretic herbs increase the discharge of urine. You might be interested to know that urinalysis has been an aid to diagnosis for centuries because so many conditions leave their signatures in urine. Early physicians not only sniffed urine, they tasted it, too.

Emetic. An emetic causes vomiting. The ancient Romans used emetics to empty their stomachs and make room for the next course during a lavish feast. Special rooms, called vomitoriums, were set aside for this purpose. If your villa wasn't equipped with a vomitorium, you were nobody in old Rome.

Emmenagogue. These substances promote menstrual discharge. There are more than a dozen useful herbs for problems connected with difficult menses.

Emollient. An emollient is similar to a demulcent. Demulcents are used internally; emollients are for external use. They are primarily used in ointments and lotions formulated to soothe and heal various skin conditions.

Expectorant. An expectorant helps the patient bring up and spit out (expectorate) phlegm that accumulates in the lungs and windpipe.

Febrifuge. Any agent that helps bring down a fever is a febrifuge. Antipyretic is another term with the same meaning.

Hepatic. An hepatic tea, as you might expect, exerts a beneficial effect on the liver and on the gallbladder as well. Agrimony, which the French drink as a tisane (tea), is considered a good liver tonic with obstruction-removing properties.

Laxative. A laxative initiates, stimulates, and increases peristaltic action. An apierient is a mild herb with gentle laxative properties. A true laxative herbal tea stimulates a bowel movement. Cathartics encourage the intestines to act and are stronger than either apierients or laxatives. Purges clean out the entire gastrointestinal tract and have a lot of power. Under the influence of a cathartic or purgative, nature won't wait for a convenient moment.

Lythontryptic. Historically, lythontryptic teas have benefited bladder complaints. The medical use of the herb uva ursi for the treatment of UTIs (urinary tract infections) dates back to the thirteenth century. This plant is mildly diuretic and is credited with being an effective disinfectant of the urinary tract.

Nervine. Nervines are used for calming the nerves. In days gone by, valerian was the apothecary's first choice as a calmative for an attack of nerves, even hysteria. In medieval times, this herb was called "all-heal" and was much prized. Watch out for this one, though; because valerian acts directly on the nervous sytem, it must be used carefully. An overdose can cause headaches, dizziness, "mirages" (hallucinations), and muscle spasms.

Oxytocic. See Parturient.

Parturient. Parturient teas intensify labor and speed childbirth. Lady's mantle and thyme are both traditional "woman's herbs." A very old herbal says of thyme tea: "Thyme is pungent and hot. It increases the flow of urine and menstruation and, in normal births, speeds delivery. A single draught cleanses the noble internal parts of the body."

Pectoral. Think "pecs" and you'll be in the right area of the body. Teas prepared with pectorals are traditionally believed to be of worth against diseases of the chest and lungs.

Potentiator. An herb that increases the action of another herb is called a potentiator.

Purgative. See Laxative.

Rubefacient. Rubefacients heat and redden the skin. They are often used as an ingredient in ointments and linaments.

Sedative. Similar to nervines, sedative teas are used to quiet and tranquilize the nervous system. Many herbs are credited with calming properties. Chamomile tea has been used to calm and soothe for centuries.

Stimulant. This term is easy; stimulants are the healing teas that are traditionally used to heat the body, raise the temperature, increase general awareness, and generally "rev" up the internal systems of the body on a quick-fix basis. The effects of stimulant teas are transitory in nature.

Stomachic. This one is easy, too. A stomachic stimulates the production of digestive juices, thereby aiding the digestive processes. It also relieves symptoms of gastric disorders.

Tonic. A tonic, like a corroborant, is an invigorating, sustaining, and strengthening tea. Old "receipts" for tonics show they are a compound-medicine composed of a variety of ingredients. In many cultures, including "American," it was considered wise to take a dose of "spring tonic."

Vulnerary. Vulneraries are plant substances that are useful in healing wounds, internal or external.

IN CONCLUSION

There is a tendency to think that because healing teas are brewed with natural ingredients, they are perfectly safe. And they are, for the most part. But please keep in mind that healing teas are very real "medicine." Herbs and plants were the original drugs. They remain powerful pharmaceuticals in their own right. Healing teas should be used with the same appropriate cautions you observe with pharmaceutical drugs. However, once you have mastered the art of brewing your own "medicine," you'll find it wonderfully satisfying to know you've taken a major step toward having control of your own well being.

If you want to carry your involvement with home-brewed medicinal teas a giant leap ahead, you'll find everything you need to know in the next chapter. The ABCs of Herb Cultivation gives you information on getting started growing, harvesting, drying, and storing the ingredients for your own home-grown healing teas.

5

The ABCs of Herb Cultivation

I n days gone by, more people cultivated their own ingredients for healing teas than shopped at the apothecary. Every family had a kitchen garden for vegetables and an herb garden for medicines and seasonings. Today, many people grow culinary herbs—sweet basil and thyme, for example—on a sunny kitchen windowsill. Plucking a few leaves of fresh basil or scissoring off a frond of pungent thyme to throw into a pot bubbling on the stove adds incomparable flavor.

In this day and age, only a lucky few have the space needed for vegetables or the time required to tend a family-sized plot. On the other hand, almost everyone has room for an herb garden, even if it's just a small space on the patio or an old bookcase next to a window. This chapter is for those of you who want to try your hand at growing, harvesting, drying, and storing your own herbs. Cultivating the medicinal plants you need to brew your own healing teas can be very rewarding, and it's easier than you think.

A HOME FOR YOUR HERBS

The traditional place for the household's herb garden has always been a sunny spot handy to the kitchen door. If you have even a tiny yard that receives sun during at least part of the day, you can easily grow a few of the medicinal herbs.

However, in today's modern world, many of us live in homes that have patios rather than yards or in high-rise apartments without a bit of land to call our own. Fortunately, some herbs are happy indoors, and you can always consider a combination of indoor and outdoor herb gardening. For instance, small potted herbs will flourish on tiered shelves in a sunny city window without ever a breath of fresh air. If you have a balcony or patio, large pots can be moved outside in the summer to catch some rays, and brought inside for shelter against winter's icy winds.

One particularly attractive method of cultivating a variety of herbs in a small place is the traditional "strawberry pot" or "strawberry barrel." Many nurseries stock various sizes of what are termed "strawberry pots." These pots, traditionally of terra cotta, have a number of "pockets" opening inside the pot and protruding slightly from its rounded outside. The pots range in size from small, with three pockets, to giant, with fifty openings (see Figure 5.1). They are very attractive when a selection of herbs is tucked into their pockets. The silvery-gray, myriad shades of green, and tiny flowering varieties of herbs are showcased against the deep-rusty orange of the terra cotta.

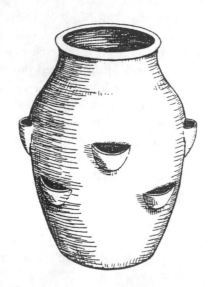

**Figure 5.1   Strawberry
Pot**

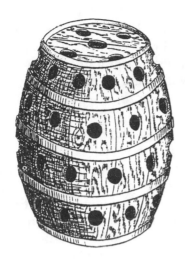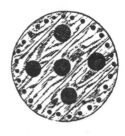

Figure 5.2   Strawberry Barrel and Lid

A "strawberry barrel," shown in Figure 5.2, has the same design and can be easily made at home. Most nurseries carry wooden barrels and half-barrels. A half-barrel can provide a home for up to 100 herbs. Half-size, three-quarter, and even one-quarter size barrels are also readily available. You can also obtain thirty-gallon whiskey casks suitable for transforming into herb barrels from many distilleries.

If the idea of fixing up a barrel as a home for your herbs appeals to you, first, secure a suitable vessel. The next step is to drill holes two inches in diameter and four inches apart (in every direction) in a pleasing pattern around the circumference of the barrel and in the lid. The lid, also seen in Figure 5.2, will probably accommodate only five or six 2-inch holes. You'll also need to drill a series of small holes around the outside circumference of the lid to provide spaces for watering. If you don't have a drill or the space to work, prevail upon a friend with a home workshop. You're sure to know someone who will think your herb barrel is a fascinating project. Promise the person some dried medicinal herbs as a barter.

GETTING READY TO PLANT

Once you have your strawberry pot, barrel, or other planter on hand, the next step is to provide a suitable growing medium for your herbs with a core or base of small rocks to provide drainage. You'll need a porous soil mix that holds water and nutrients but drains quickly. Ask the nursery staff for a good, commercial potting soil that is light, uniform in texture, disease-free (sterilized), and nutritionally balanced.

If you have decided to put your herb garden in a barrel and the holes are drilled, here's how to fill the barrel: Begin by making a mound of small rocks in the center of the barrel. Next, pour soil into the barrel around and as high as the mound of rocks. You may wish to dampen the potting soil to prevent it from spilling out the drilled holes, but don't worry if the soil and rocks intermingle where they meet. Continue piling rocks in the center and soil around the circumference until the entire barrel has been well filled.

If you want to help hasten the inevitable settling of the soil and you happen to have a muscle-man handy, have him lift the barrel a few inches and let it drop several times. Otherwise, water the filled barrel well and wait a few days before planting to allow gravity to take care of the job. If you plant before everything has had time to settle, you may find your tender young herbs out of position and hanging by the neck (until dead) out of their respective holes.

Consider the water requirements of your herbs when positioning them in the barrel. Plants that need a lot of moisture should be positioned in the lid itself or in the top half of the barrel. Those requiring less moisture will be quite happy in the lower half of the barrel. Generally speaking, most herbs are drought-resistant and don't mind being on the dry side. Container-grown herbs that are correctly potted in a good porous mixture with good drainage can be watered freely with little danger of root rot.

THE GROWING MEDIUM

Remember that a good potting soil for herbs (or any container-grown plant) should be light in texture and porous enough to insure good drainage and an adequate oxygen supply. It should hold a lot of water and nutrients without becoming compacted around tender roots, but shouldn't retain moisture so long that root rot can develop. The pH and nutrient content should be balanced and the mix must be disease-free to insure healthy plants.

If you're really getting into this and want to get your plants off to a healthy start, the following recipe will yield an excellent potting soil:

Super-Charged Potting Soil*

15 parts (shovels, buckets, or any container
measured by volume) topsoil
5 parts horticultural grade vermiculite or peat moss

To "charge" 10 cubic feet of the soil, add:

6.5 cups cottonseed meal
6.5 cups compost or dairy manure
1 teaspoon seawood meal

*Adapted from *Super Nutrition Gardening* by Dr. William S. Peavy and Warren Peary (Avery Publishing Group, Garden City Park, New York, 1992).

SELECTING THE PLANTS

Like all plants, herbs are classified according to their life cycle in the natural state. For example, annuals must be planted every year, unless their growing conditions are such that they seed themselves. Biennials should be planted every year, too. Biennials put forth only leaves their first year. You have to wait for the second year for flowers. By planting biennials every year, you'll always have a supply of flowers to harvest.

Perennials are those obliging plants that last for many years with a minimum of care. Perennials are quite often arranged in the center of a garden and left to fend for themselves, while the annuals and biennials are grouped around the outside perimeter, making it easier to reset them every year.

If you are planning a small trial-planting of herbs, consider selecting from among the premiere medicinal herbs: calendula, chamomile, dandelion, echinacea, horsetail, mallow, mullein, sage, and St. John's wort. These herbs and others are discussed in Chapter 6, A Selection of Natural Medicinals, where you will find a brief description of the healing plant, including how tall it grows and its favorite habitat. For some reason, this vital information is often missing in published material on herbal medicine. Although the information on growth patterns is not complete, the general guidelines given for each plant will help you decide what herbs will do well given the climate and space in your garden.

If you decide to start from scratch, the seed packets you purchase will give you detailed growing instructions. For the most part, seeds are started indoors in a flat container. All you need to do is keep the soil moist by misting it daily, baby the tiny sprouts along, and move them to their permanent home when they have achieved a suitable size.

Getting started is even easier if you buy young, potted herbs in a nursery. Don't be afraid to ask questions. A knowledgeable staff member will certainly be happy to pass on his enthusiasm and will tell you how to care for your new botanicals.

Once the herbs are growing, you'll need to know when and how to gather them for your medicine closet.

HARVESTING

Whether you are harvesting herbs for immediate use in their fresh state or for drying, they should be gathered at the time in their growing cycle when they are most potent. If you are harvesting the whole plant, it should be gathered early in the growing cycle when it is just coming into bloom. Fruits and berries should be harvested only when they become fully ripe. Flowers should be gathered when they are in full bloom but are still quite young and fresh. Flowers are most potent during the beginning of flowering. Leaves should be taken when they are still quite young, but they must be fully developed. Leaves are most vigorous just before the buds open, but also may be taken during flowering. Collect only roots that are strong and fully developed, not stringy or fragile. Roots should be dug out only when the plant is dormant, either early spring or late fall.

It's best to gather the medicinal plants no earlier than mid-morning on a sunny day. There are two reasons for this. First, you want to give the sun time to dry the moisture that has accumulated overnight in the form of dew. Second, plants that have been warmed by the sun are in their most potent state. The volatile oils are free-flowing and strongest when the plants are warm. As a general rule of thumb, it's best to schedule your harvest time from around 10 o'clock in the morning to around 3 o'clock in the afternoon.

You will, of course, select only clean, healthy plants that show no insect infestation: no chewed leaves, mites on the underside of leaves, or ragged blossoms. If you are gathering in the field, and not your own garden, bypass roadsides and highways where the plants have been polluted by passing traffic. Herbs growing near railway embankments, dirty streams, or industrial plants are obviously unsuitable for harvesting. Fields, meadows, woodlands, and pastures are usually excellent sources of healing tea ingredients. Watch out for grazing land that may have been chemically fertilized by a farmer anxious to provide good grasses for his stock.

Please be as considerate when field-gathering as you are when harvesting in your own garden. Don't pull plants out by their roots and don't leave a mess behind you. Always leave several plants of a given species to insure sufficient growth for future harvests. When gathering leaves and blossoms only, snip them off between your fingernails to minimize damage to the plant. Pinching is preferable to cutting because the pinch acts to close the broken stem and helps seal in the plant's vital juices. You may, when necessary, scissor tough stems when gathering the entire herb, but leave at least one strong growing stem so the plant can heal itself. If you are gathering roots, please dig them out carefully. When possible, divide the root clump and replant a portion of it to insure future growth.

The time-honored method of carrying herbs home is to layer them loosely in an open basket. There's a reason for this. You must take care not to crush delicate blossoms and leaves. If the leaves and blossoms are crushed and the stems are broken, some of the vital oils can escape, reducing the herb's medicinal properties.

If you don't have a basket handy, use a brown paper bag. Don't ever carry your prizes home in plastic. Harmful condensation will form as the plants sweat inside the plastic. You may not even notice that any damage has been done until the drying process has been completed and the herbs turn black, rendering them useless for healing teas.

DRYING

Unless you are going to immediately brew a healing tea, it's necessary to dry the natural medicinals to stop the natural fermentation that would otherwise occur. Plan to dry your herbs and herb parts as soon as they are harvested. Don't wait. Drying preserves the healing agents you want in your healing teas. The drying process also insures that any fungi or bacteria are destroyed. Whole herbs selected for drying should not be washed.

When drying the entire plant, tie several stems together loosely and hang the bunch upside down in a warm, airy place until thoroughly dry. When drying leaves and flowers, spread them out in a single layer and space them well apart so they don't touch each other. It is best to lay them on a fine mesh screen that allows air to circulate all around the herb parts. You can also use a white cloth or unprinted paper. Butcher paper, shelf lining paper (unprinted and unglazed), even brown paper bags opened up and pressed flat are all suitable.

Roots, barks, or thick, fleshy herb parts may be dried in a very slow oven (no higher than 100°F) to hasten the process. If you have a gas oven, the pilot flame alone will often provide sufficient heat. Roots should be scrubbed clean of soil, but don't wash bark or thick tuberous herb parts. Cut roots in half lengthwise, sliver bark lengthwise with the grain, and slice any thick herbs into smaller segments to help them dry faster and more evenly.

On warm summer days, you may dry herb parts outdoors, but not in direct sunlight. The only drawback to using summer's heat to accomplish the drying process is that the herbs must be brought indoors overnight to guard against their gathering moisture.

Any warm, well-ventilated room provides a suitable environment for drying herbs. Unless your herb parts are drying in the oven with the door closed, the kitchen isn't suitable. Cooking odors can permeate the plants. The laundry room isn't suitable either because it's usually full of steamy, moisture-laden air. An attic is first choice, but not many people have attics anymore. A spare room or unused bedroom will do very well.

STORING DRIED HERBS

Before storing dried ingredients for healing teas, test them to make sure the herb parts are thoroughly dry. Fully dried parts will break easily or powder when snapped between your fingers. Store your dried herbs in glass jars or small boxes that can be made airtight. Green or amber jars that protect your precious herbs from light are best. Keep the containers in a dark, dry cupboard and the medicinal properties will be protected throughout the winter.

There are two "don'ts" to remember when storing the ingredients for brewing healing teas. First, don't use plastic or metal containers. Second, don't be greedy. You can't keep vast quantities of herbs on hand and expect them to last for years. Dried herbs lose quality as time passes. They should be used within six to eight months for best results.

Fortunately, Mother Nature is ever obliging. A new selection of annual herbs is as close as your local nursery. Even better, if you have planted perennials, green, growing herbs will thrust up their green shoots every spring, as they have done since time began.

Once your herbs are happily settled and well established, their subtle colors will enhance any corner and their faint fragrances will freshen the air. In addition, you will be rewarded with fresh cuttings of your favorite medicinals just about any time of the year. The first cup of healing tea you brew from your own homegrown herbs can be a thrilling experience.

IN CONCLUSION

Of course, you'll want to know the natural medicinals that work best for what ails you at any given moment. Just turn the page; my pharmacopoeia for you is about to unfold.

Part II
Selecting Teas

. . . and the leaf thereof for medicine.

Ezekiel 47:12

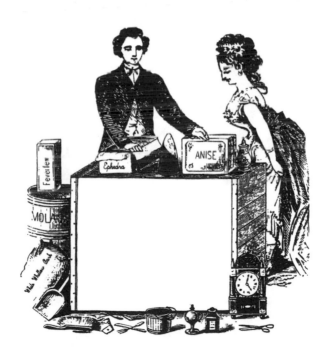

6

A Selection of Natural Medicinals for Brewing Healing Teas

In this section, you will find an alphabetical listing of natural medicinals. Most—but not all—of these medicinals are beneficial herbs that have traditionally been used in the brewing of healing teas. This is not an encyclopedic list, but encompasses those herbs I have found I reach for most often to ease the complaints and health problems that arise in the day-to-day running of a busy household.

In order to identify the herbs and other natural medicinals that are best for your condition, consult Table 6.1, which lists common disorders and the herbs used to treat them. This A to Z trouble-shooting guide includes some very serious health problems such as cancer. Several natural medicinals have been used throughout history to treat cancer, but that doesn't mean you should ignore your doctor and rely solely on teas. On the other hand, if you have arthritis, choose one of the beneficial herbs listed next to "arthritis" in the table, find that herb in the alphabetical listing, and follow the guidelines for its use. You can also check out the other ancient herbs that have been used successfully for centuries to treat the problem. Whatever disorder you may have, remember that healing teas may bring you some ease, but they must not be used without your doctor's

Table 6.1   A to Z Trouble-Shooting Guide

Condition	Beneficial Herbs
Acne	Bee pollen, burdock, dandelion, echinacea, ginseng, gotu kola, propolis, sarsaparilla
Adrenal-function-related problems	Astragalus, ginseng, licorice, lobelia, mahuang
Age-related disorders	Bee pollen, ginkgo, gotu kola, sage, yerba mate
AIDS	Astragalus, bee pollen, echinacea, garlic, ginseng, goldenseal, pau d'arco, red clover, St. John's wort, taheebo, yerba mate
Alcoholism	Angelica, capsicum, chamomile, skullcap
Allergies	Angelica, bee pollen, echinacea, garlic, licorice, mahuang, mullein, pau d'arco, yerba mate
Anemia	Dandelion
Arthritis	Alfalfa, black cohosh, burdock, capsicum, chamomile, feverfew, garlic, ginkgo, licorice, mullein, pau d'arco, red clover, sarsaparilla, valerian, yerba mate
Asthma	Alfalfa, black cohosh, capsicum, chamomile, garlic, ginkgo, goldenseal, horehound, lobelia, mahuang, marshmallow, mullein
Bed-wetting	Damiana, pau d'arco, St. John's wort
Blood-pressure-related problems	Bee pollen, black cohosh, capsicum, dandelion, garlic, gotu kola, green tea, ginseng (Siberian)
Blood purifiers	Alfalfa, bee pollen, burdock, dandelion, garlic, goldenseal, gotu kola, pau d'arco, red clover, rose hips, sarsaparilla, yerba mate
Bone-related problems	Comfrey (for external use only), dandelion, horsetail, red raspberry
Bronchitis	Angelica, licorice, lobelia, mahuang, mullein, St. John's wort
Burns	Calendula, comfrey (for external use only), propolis
Cancer	Bee pollen, cascara sagrada, dandelion, echinacea, Essiac, garlic, ginseng, goldenseal, green tea, pau d'arco, propolis
Cholesterol-related problems	Bee pollen, black cohosh, dandelion, garlic
Circulatory-system-related problems	Angelica, capsicum, dong quai, garlic, gingko, ginger, licorice, mahuang, skullcap, valerian
Cold extremities	Angelica, capsicum, peppermint

Condition	Beneficial Herbs
Colds and flu	Angelica, anise, black cohosh, capsicum, chamomile, echinacea, garlic, ginger, ginseng, goldenseal, green tea, horehound, licorice, lobelia, mahuang, red raspberry, rose hips, sage, spearmint, valerian
Colic	Anise, echinacea, ginger, peppermint, valerian
Colon toxicity	Alfalfa, bee pollen, cascara sagrada, chamomile, ginger, goldenseal, horsetail, licorice, marshmallow, psyllium
Congestion	Black cohosh, comfrey (for external use only), feverfew, ginger, horehound, licorice, mahuang, mullein, St. John's wort
Constipation	Cascara sagrada, licorice, psyllium
Coughs	Angelica, anise, black cohosh, goldenseal, horehound, licorice, lobelia, marshmallow, pau d'arco, rose hips
Dandruff	Sage, spearmint
Dental-related problems	Goldenseal, green tea, parsley, propolis, red raspberry, sage
Depression	Bee pollen, ginkgo, ginseng, gotu kola, licorice, St. John's wort
Diabetes	Alfalfa, capsicum, garlic, ginseng, goldenseal, pau d'arco
Diarrhea	Licorice, marshmallow, peppermint, red raspberry, sage
Digestion-related problems	Alfalfa, angelica, anise, bee pollen, burdock, capsicum, chamomile, dandelion, garlic, ginger, goldenseal, horsetail, licorice, marshmallow, parsley, peppermint, sage, sarsaparilla, saw palmetto, spearmint, wintergreen
Ear-related problems	Calendula, ginkgo, goldenseal, horsetail, mahuang, mullein (flower)
Epilepsy	Lobelia
Eye-related problems	Eyebright, ginkgo, horsetail
Fatigue, mental	Ginkgo, gotu kola, sage, yerba mate
Fatigue, physical	Astragalus, bee pollen, damiana, garlic, ginkgo, ginseng, gotu kola, mahuang, red clover, sarsaparilla, yerba mate
Female disorders	Angelica, bee pollen, black cohosh, calendula, chamomile, damiana, dong quai, feverfew, ginger, licorice, parsley, red raspberry, St. John's wort, uva ursi
Fever	Calendula, chamomile, feverfew, lobelia, red raspberry, sarsaparilla, white willow bark
Flatulence	See Gas.

Condition	Beneficial Herbs
Gallbladder-related problems	Cascara sagrada, licorice
Gallstones	Cascara sagrada, parsley
Gastrointestinal problems	Cascara sagrada, dandelion, ginger, licorice, marshmallow, psyllium, sarsaparilla
Gas	Angelica, anise, ginger, horehound, parsley, peppermint, spearmint, wintergreen
Gout	Burdock, dandelion, red clover, sarsaparilla
Hair-related problems	Bee pollen, horsetail, parsley, sage, sarsaparilla
Headache	Chamomile, damiana, feverfew, peppermint, skullcap, St. John's wort, valerian, white willow bark, wintergreen, yerba mate
Headache, migraine	Capsicum, feverfew, uva ursi, white willow bark
Heartburn	Angelica, ginger, peppermint
Heart problems	Angelica, bee pollen, capsicum, garlic, goldenseal, ginkgo, gotu kola, green tea, licorice, lobelia, skullcap, uva ursi, valerian
Hemorrhoids	Burdock, calendula, cascara sagrada, chamomile, goldenseal, psyllium, uva ursi
High blood pressure	See Blood-pressure-related problems.
Hypoglycemia	Dandelion, licorice
Immune-function-related problems	Astragalus, bee pollen, burdock, echinacea, garlic, ginseng, goldenseal, licorice, pau d'arco, propolis, yerba mate
Infection	Bee pollen, echinacea, garlic, goldenseal, gotu kola, licorice, pau d'arco, propolis, red clover, rose hips
Insect bites and stings	Black cohosh, calendula, burdock, sage, St. John's wort
Insomnia	Chamomile, mullein, skullcap, St. John's wort, valerian
Joint pain	Capsicum, feverfew, ginger, lobelia, marshmallow, white willow bark, wintergreen
Kidney-related problems	Astragalus, capsicum, dandelion, ginkgo, ginger, goldenseal, horsetail, mahuang, milk thistle, rose hips, sarsaparilla, spearmint, uva ursi
Lethargy	Astragalus, damiana, dandelion, echinacea, dong quai, ginseng, goldenseal
Lice	Angelica

Condition	Beneficial Herbs
Liver-related problems	Alfalfa, cascara sagrada, chamomile, dandelion, feverfew, garlic, goldenseal, gotu kola, horehound, licorice, milk thistle, pau d'arco, propolis, sarsaparilla, uva ursi
Low blood pressure	See Blood-pressure-related problems.
Lung-related problems	Angelica, astragalus, capsicum, ginkgo, ginseng, goldenseal, lobelia, mahuang, marshmallow, mullein, parsley, pau d'arco, red clover
Male disorders	Bee pollen, damiana, dong quai, echinacea, ginseng, propolis, sarsaparilla, saw palmetto
Migraine	See Headache, migraine.
Motion sickness	Anise, ginger
Muscle cramps	Comfrey (for external use only), chamomile
Nail-related problems	Bee pollen, horsetail, red raspberry
Nausea	Anise, capsicum, ginger, licorice, peppermint
Nervous-system-related problems	Chamomile, damiana, dong quai, gingko, gotu kola, rose hips, skullcap, sarsaparilla, St. John's wort, valerian, yerba mate
Night sweats	Black cohosh, sage
Nursing-related problems	Anise, red raspberry
Pain	Capsicum, chamomile, comfrey (for external use only), feverfew, mullein, skullcap, valerian, white willow bark
Pancreas-related problems	Dandelion, goldenseal, uva ursi
Rheumatism	Alfalfa, angelica, black cohosh, capsicum, chamomile, dandelion, gotu kola, horsetail, pau d'arco, peppermint, sarsaparilla, skullcap, white willow bark, wintergreen
Sex-related problems	Bee pollen, damiana, ginseng, gotu kola, saw palmetto
Sinusitis	Anise, black cohosh, echinacea, garlic, goldenseal, horehound, mahuang, mullein
Skin conditions	Angelica, bee pollen, calendula, burdock, echinacea, goldenseal, gotu kola, horsetail, licorice, milk thistle, red clover, red raspberry, rose hips, sarsaparilla, St. John's wort, wintergreen
Smoking, problems quitting	Lobelia

Condition	Beneficial Herbs
Sore throat	Ginger, goldenseal, horehound, lobelia, licorice, mullein, propolis, wintergreen
Spasms and tics	Ginger, licorice, lobelia, peppermint, skullcap, valerian
Spleen-related problems	Capsicum, dandelion, ginger
Stress	See Fatique, mental; Depression.
Stroke	Preventives: capsicum, ginkgo, gotu kola, green tea
Ulcers	Alfalfa, calendula, capsicum, comfrey (for external use only), garlic, ginseng, goldenseal, licorice, marshmallow, pau d'arco, peppermint, valerian
Urinary-tract-related problems	Alfalfa, chamomile, dandelion, goldenseal, gotu kola, horsetail, parsley, rose hips, saw palmetto, uva ursi
Varicose veins	Calendula, capsicum, goldenseal
Venereal diseases	Sarsaparilla
Vomiting	Ginger
Water retention	Angelica, anise, astragalus, dandelion, gotu kola, horsetail, mahuang, parsley, uva ursi, yerba mate
Weight control	Astragalus, bee pollen, mahuang, parsley, peppermint, red clover, yerba mate
Wounds	Comfrey (for external use only), goldenseal, horsetail, propolis
Yeast infections	Echinacea, garlic, goldenseal, pau d'arco, propolis, wintergreen

permission and should never be used instead of prescribed medication.

When brewing the teas, remember that most herbs produce a bland brew. However, you may find some teas quite unpleasant tasting. It doesn't matter. The herbs listed here brew into true *medicinals*. It's not a good idea to add a little sugar to "help the medicine go down." Anything you add has the potential to change the chemical properties of the brew and may dilute its usefulness as a healing tea. If you absolutely must tinker with the taste, stir in a spoonful of raw honey only, nothing else.

THE NIFTY FIFTY-FOUR:
AN ALPHABETICAL LISTING OF NATURAL MEDICINALS

The natural medicinals reviewed in the following pages—fifty-four in all—have been selected because they have withstood the test of time. Over the centuries, all these medicinals have racked up solid empirical evidence of their health benefits. Many of these items from the natural world have been investigated by scientists as well as health-care practitioners. Most have earned solid support from well-informed medical detectives around the globe.

If you will take the time to become acquainted with the many wonders available in nature's pharmacy, I know the healing teas will be as helpful to you and your family as they have been to mine.

Alfalfa *(Medicago sativa)*

This alkaline herb is a well-known detoxifier with anti-inflammatory properties. It sweetens the stomach and is especially helpful for cleansing the liver. Alfalfa fights colon disorders, urinary tract infections and ulcers. A cup of alfalfa tea daily may bring relief from rheumatoid arthritis. Because it enhances pituitary function, alfalfa has long been used against diabetes.

DESCRIPTION AND PARTS USED

Alfalfa is primarily known in the United States as superior cattle fodder (which it is). This leguminous plant from Europe has attractive bluish-purple flowers. Almost all of this herb—leaves, petals, flowers, and sprouts—has medicinal properties. Only the roots are not used.

HISTORICAL NOTES

Alfalfa was called the "father of all foods" by the ancient Arabs who considered it a highly nutritious legume. In 1597, the English master herbalist John Gerard recommended alfalfa for upset stomach. Natural healers have long followed that advice. Because it is a natural anti-inflammatory agent, alfalfa has been used against arthritis.

SCIENTIFIC FINDINGS

The leaves of alfalfa are especially rich in minerals, including calcium, magnesium, potassium, and beta carotene, as well as eight essential amino acids, chlorophyll, and the vitamins A, B complex, C, D, E, and K.

TRADITIONAL USE

To prepare a natural detoxifier and mild diuretic, brew a healing tea using 1 tablespoon (1/2 ounce or 12 grams) of the dried herb. Follow the general directions given in Chapter 3.

CONSIDERATIONS

Alfalfa has been known to aggravate autoimmune disorders. Do not give alfalfa in any instance where there is an impaired immune system.

Angelica
(*Angelica atropurpurea*)

Angelica is credited with being a stimulant that has carminative (inducing expulsion of gas) and antispasmodic properties. Since ancient times, angelica tea has been given to rheumatics and those who suffer from cold hands and feet because it helps stimulate blood flow. As an antispasmodic, angelica fights PMS and menstrual cramps. Angelica is a time-honored expectorant (promoting expulsion) that fights bronchitis, loosens phlegm, and helps make seasonal allergies more bearable.

DESCRIPTION AND PARTS USED

Angelica atropurpurea is a biennial with purplish stems and large green-tinged white flowers that appear during its second year of growth. It flourishes in rich loamy soil and loves moist bottom-lands, where it can attain a height of five or six feet. The medicinal

Sweet Angelica

The stalks of Angelica are sometimes candied by simmering them in a heavy sugar syrup until they absorb all the sugar they can hold. After drying, the candied Angelica is ready to eat. This old confection was much enjoyed in ancient times and is still considered a treat today.

properties of this striking plant are most concentrated in the seeds and root, although the stalk and leaves are sometimes used.

HISTORICAL NOTES

Legend has it that the garden variety of angelica—*angelica archangelica*—was named after the Archangel Raphael, who was so touched by this pious act that he revealed the secrets of the herb to the French monk who had so honored him. Henceforth, angelica was used to ease the suffering of plague victims.

The master herbalists of old considered angelica a most versatile medicinal. In the Middle Ages, the oft-quoted Culpeper wrote, "Angelica is of especial use in swounings, tremblings and passions of the heart, soothes a feeble stomach, to expell any windy or noysome vapours from it. It helpeth the pleurisy, as well as all other diseases of the lungs and breast."

It may surprise you to learn that the ancient Chinese medicinal dong quai (see page 123), often called "woman's ginseng," is also a species of angelica.

SCIENTIFIC FINDINGS

Much of the research on *Angelica atropurpurea*, as is so often the case, has centered on extracts of the plant, rather than on isolated constituents. Various pharmacological properties have been scientifically identified including antibacterial activity, muscle-relaxing effects, allergy-modulating abilities, and tonic and pain-relieving qualities.

The Golden Drink
of the Angels

You may be familiar with Frangelica, a liqueur flavored with angelica. The Swiss have a traditional recipe for angelica liqueur, which they call Vespetro. Traditionally, it has been used as a warming and stimulating medicinal liqueur. Just a small sip of Vespetro is said to quickly relieve cramps, chills, digestive upsets, and flatulence. Even though it tastes delicious, this is a true medicinal tincture, not an after-dinner liqueur. The recommended dose of the "golden drink of the angels" is ten drops in water, taken three times daily thirty minutes before meals. Here's a modification of an old Swiss recipe:

2 ounces Angelica seeds
1/4 ounce anise seeds
1/4 ounce fennel seeds
1/5 ounce coriander seeds (approximate)
8 ounces of food-grade alcoholic spirits such as vodka
(Do not use rubbing alcohol.)
1 pound fine sugar
2 1/2 pints pure water

1. *Grind the seeds together. If you want to follow tradition, use a mortar and pestle. If your kitchen boasts a seed mill, that will make it much easier to do the job.*

2. *Have ready a glass bottle holding the food-grade alcoholic spirits. Vodka is the best choice, because it has so little flavor of its own. Add the well-pulverized and blended seeds to the vodka, cork the bottle well, and give it a good shake.*

3. *Allow the mixture to stand in a warm place for 8 days to steep. Shake it every time you think about it. After 8 days of steeping, strain the mixture through a cheesecloth bag, twisting well to extract every drop.*

4. *Dissolve the sugar in the water. Blend in the flavored spirits. Bottle and cork tightly.*

TRADITIONAL USE

Internal. Following the guidelines given in Chapter 3, prepare an infusion by pouring eight ounces of freshly boiled water over 1 heaping teaspoon (1/6 ounce or 4 grams) of angelica root. The usual dose is 2 or 3 tablespoons of tea taken three times daily.

External. To ease the aches and pains of rheumatic joints, prepare an angelica poultice following the directions given in Chapter 3. Apply as hot as the patient can tolerate. Reheat the herbs and replace as the poultice cools. For body lice, prepare a strong wash (see Chapter 3) and bathe the affected areas. Angelica will get rid of the pests and relieve the itching at the same time.

CONSIDERATIONS

Angelica is a powerful emmenagogue (induces menstrual flow). It must not be used by pregnant women. Also, because angelica has the potential to increase sugar in the urine, diabetics and hypoglycemics should avoid this herb. Large doses of angelica can affect blood pressure, heart action, and breathing. Do not exceed the recommended dose.

Anise *(Pimpinella anisum)*

Anise is a diuretic (increases urine) and carminative herb, useful for expelling gas, eliminating colic, relieving abdominal pain, sweetening a sour stomach, preventing nausea, and improving digestion. Anise soothes a hacking cough, helps clear congestion, and relieves cold symptoms. When taken by nursing mothers, it stimulates and improves milk production, and may—with just a few sips—help ease a colicky baby. When permitted to dissolve in the mouth, anise candy fights motion sickness.

DESCRIPTION AND PARTS USED

Anise is an ancient, much-valued herb that makes a lovely garden plant. It is remarkably easy to grow, although the seeds must be kept around 70°F to insure germination. Anise doesn't like to be moved, so sow the seeds where you want the plant to live.

An annual, anise reaches a height of eighteen to twenty-four inches. The first leaves are large and wide; the secondary leaves that come later are featherlike. By midsummer, tiny clusters of yellowish-white flowers appear, followed in late summer by green seeds. When the seeds ripen and turn grayish-brown, they're ready for harvest. It's the sweet and spicy seeds, tasting faintly of licorice, that hold the medicinal qualities of this herb.

HISTORICAL NOTES

In Gerard's herbal, the old master had this to say about anise: "The seed wasteth and consumeth winde, is good against belchings, and upbraidings of the stomacke, allayeth gripings of the belly, provoketh urine gently, maketh abundance of milke, and stirreth up bodily lust . . . " Although anise was once considered an aphrodisiac, Gerard was mistaken; it does not "stir up bodily lust" in the slightest. However, Gerard was correct when he wrote: "The same being dried by the fire and taken with honey clenseth the brest very much from flegmaticke superfluities and, if it be taken with bitter almonds, it doth helpe the old cough." Even earlier, Hippocrates had recommended anise for coughs and sour stomachs. It is still valued for these properties today.

SCIENTIFIC FINDINGS

Analysis shows that anise contains several B vitamins, choline, calcium, iron, potassium, and magnesium. Some studies indicate anise contains plant hormones that are similar to estrogen; this may explain why the seeds are recommended for nursing mothers.

TRADITIONAL USE

Internal. To brew a healing tea of anise, pour 8 ounces of freshly boiled water over 2 or 3 teaspoons of anise seeds, well bruised, "slightly crushed" in the parlance of the herbalist. Steep for 8 minutes, strain well, sweeten to taste with honey, if you like, and sip hot. If the seeds are not well bruised, you'll need to prepare a decoction to extract their medicinal qualities. (Full directions for preparing teas [infusions] and decoctions can be found in Chapter 3.)

CONSIDERATIONS

Anise seed has been used for centuries with no reports of toxicity. It is so mild that small sips of brewed tea have been given to colicky babies with no ill effects.

Astragalus *(Astragalus membranaceous)*

Astragalus, pronounced ah-strag-ah-lus, enhances immune function, aids adrenal gland function, strengthens weak lungs, and is considered an excellent tonic tea that tones up the entire system. It increases metabolic function, promotes healing, and energizes tired glands. Because astragalus has diuretic properties, it is helpful in reducing edema, especially if the kidneys are involved.

DESCRIPTION AND PARTS USED

Astragalus can attain a height of from two to five feet by its second year of growth. This plant has long oval leaves with a feathery appearance. It puts forth handsome bell-shaped flowers with pale yellow petals. The root, which has a faintly sweet taste and is the repository of the medicinal properties, is long and flexible with a wrinkled brown skin. When the dark skin is peeled away, a yellowish-white interior is revealed.

HISTORICAL NOTES

For centuries, Chinese herbalists have used a tea brewed of astragalus for a wide variety of ailments, including diabetes, heart disease, weak lungs, and high blood pressure. Because this herb is a natural diuretic, it is especially valuable in reducing water buildup in the tissues.

SCIENTIFIC FINDINGS

Studies published in Chinese medical journals show that astragalus helps activate the immune system, thereby strengthening the body's ability to fight off infections and disease. Research conducted at the

University of Texas (Houston) showed that an extract of this herb helps strengthen impaired immune function in cancer patients undergoing chemotherapy and radiation treatments.

TRADITIONAL USE

Internal. Because the medicinal properties of astragalus are stored in the root, it's necessary to prepare a decoction according to the directions given in Chapter 3. Take 1 to 3 cups of tea daily as needed to help boost the defensive forces of the body and restore energies lost due to illness.

CONSIDERATIONS

Patients undergoing treatment for cancer should not take astragalus or any other medicinal, natural or otherwise, without the approval of their physicians.

Bee Pollen

Honeybee pollen has been used for centuries as both food and medicine. It is called the "world's only perfect food" because quality blended bee pollen contains every nutrient the human body requires. Bee pollen is a champion energizer that fights fatigue, combats cancer, eliminates depression, stimulates the reproductive systems of both men and women, and eases digestive and colon disorders. It has documented antibiotic, antiviral, antiseptic, and antifungal properties.

DESCRIPTION AND PARTS USED

Honeybee pollen is gathered by honeybees from the hearts of flowers. Microscopic flecks of flower pollen are moistened with honey by the harvesting bee, packed into pellets in the "pollen baskets" on the bee's rear legs, and carried home to the hive. When pollen traps are fitted on the hives, a portion of the golden granules drops through a mesh screen into a drawer for harvesting by the beekeeper.

The Perfect Snack: Honeybee Pollen Candy

Bee pollen granules taste tart and sweet and pungent all at once. They are as aromatic as the flowers in which they originate. My family relishes bee pollen, but it is an acquired taste. In case you decide bee pollen isn't quite your "cup of tea," here's a recipe for bee pollen "candy" guaranteed to change your mind. It is reprinted with permission from Royden Brown's "Bee Hive Product Bible" in which the author says it was developed by his daughter. Kids especially like this "candy," and mothers approve it as a healthy and nutritious snack.

Yield: 18 pieces

1/2 cup bee pollen granules
2 tablespoons carob powder
2 tablespoons water
3 tablespoons raw honey
1/2 cup crunchy peanut butter

1. *Put the bee pollen granules in a mixing bowl. Dissolve the powdered carob in the water and stir into the bee pollen.*

2. *Add the raw honey and mix well.*

3. *Add the peanut butter and mix thoroughly.*

4. *Using a melon baller (or your hands), form little balls from the mixture. Store the candy balls, which will remain soft, in the refrigerator.*

The fresh granules make a highly nutritious food supplement; they are also powdered and put into tablets and capsules and used in combination formulas. Because it is such a powerhouse of nutrients, bee pollen is known as the "vitamin/mineral/more" supplement.

HISTORICAL NOTES

All the products of the beehive—bee pollen, propolis (a resinlike

More From the Hive:
Balm of Gilead Salve

Here's an item of interest—a "receipt" of great-grandmother's so ancient, it's mentioned in the Bible.

As its "family" name suggests, balm of Gilead (Commiphora opobalsamum), yields a fragrant balsam, a type of oleoresin used externally that heals, soothes, and restores. This salve is considered an excellent remedy for chapped hands and lips, minor sores and cuts, frostbite, and even piles (hemorrhoids).

1 pint balm of Gilead buds
1 pint rendered fat (lard)
4 ounces mutton tallow
3 ounces honey
3 ounces beeswax
1 ounce soft soap
1 ounce colophony (rosin)
1 ounce potash (alum)

1. *Put balm of Gilead buds in a kettle with rendered fat. Boil slowly for half an hour, stirring often. Strain out the exhausted buds.*

2. *Add mutton tallow, honey, beeswax, soft soap, colophony, and potash. Continue cooking slowly until done, usually from thirty to sixty minutes, stirring often.*

substance used with beeswax in the construction of hives), royal jelly (a substance secreted by worker bees that is food for the queen bee), and honey—have been stockpiled since primitive times to tide the population over in times of famine. Many notable healers of ages past, including Hippocrates and Pliny, recommended bee pollen for a variety of ailments. Considering the broad range of beneficial properties of all the products of the hive, it's not surprising to find that the holy writings of many civilizations call the honeybee and her products especially blessed.

SCIENTIFIC FINDINGS

The anticarcinogenic (cancer-fighting) properties of bee pollen have been documented in many studies around the globe, including one conducted by William Robinson, M.D., of the United States Food and Drug Administration (FDA). European clinics that use the products of the beehive as the sole method of treatment have shown time after time that bee pollen is effective against a host of ailments, including depression, intestinal distubances, prostate problems, sexual dysfunction, and many of the so-called age-related conditions that plague society.

TRADITIONAL USE

Internal. Because heat destroys its vital enzyme activity and lowers the nutrient value of bee pollen, it does not lend itself to the brewing of a healing tea. If you wish to experience this energizer for yourself, try sprinkling the fresh granules on your morning cereal or afternoon cup of yogurt. When crushed and laced with cinnamon, powdered granules can add a delightful spiciness to any unheated food—applesauce, for example.

CONSIDERATIONS

Although the majority of people find bee pollen amazingly beneficial, a very few (.05% according to the experts) may experience a reaction to bee pollen. Begin slowly by allowing one or two granules to dissolve in your mouth. Discontinue at once if you begin wheezing or develop a rash.

Black Cohosh *(Cimicifuga racemosa)*

Black cohosh relieves sinusitis and asthma by reducing congestion and mucous buildup; it eases coughing spasms, too. This herb helps bring down cholesterol levels, regulates blood pressure, combats rheumatic pain, and helps ease some forms of arthritis. Black cohosh is also a traditional remedy for hot flashes and menstrual cramps. Used externally, black cohosh—sometimes called bugbane—reduces the irritation of insect bites by working to neutralize any poisonous residue.

DESCRIPTION AND PARTS USED

This pretty native American plant is a cousin to the buttercup. A perennial that makes a showy backdrop for smaller herbs, it is an excellent addition to an outdoor garden. Each plant produces a long stalk that divides itself into several branches; each branch bears long plumelike clusters of strong-smelling white flowers. The root is the repository of the medicinal constituents.

HISTORICAL NOTES

Native Americans were using black cohosh to bring down rheumatic swellings and reduce joint pain long before the colonists arrived. Black cohosh is considered the herbalist's "specific" against asthma, bronchitis, chronic coughs—even whooping cough.

For centuries, black cohosh has been considered a premiere "women's herb" against all sorts of female complaints, including menstrual cramps and change-of-life symptoms. It was often used to bring on labor.

SCIENTIFIC FINDINGS

Scientists have discovered that black cohosh contains an estrogen-like substance. This finding may explain why the herb has traditionally been used to treat so many female disorders. Black cohosh also contains two fatty acids (oleic and palmitic), phosphorus, tannin, vitamins A and B, and actaeine, cimicifungin, and isoferulic acid (a type of iron).

TRADITIONAL USE

Internal. Using the general directions given in Chapter 3, brew a decoction. Take 1 cup of tea twice daily to reduce the pain and swelling of rheumatic and arthritic joints. To relieve menstrual cramps, lessen hot flashes, and help relieve change-of-life symptoms, take 1 cup of tea twice daily. Do not take black cohosh longer than 3 days in a row.

External. Prepare a wash according to the general directions given in Chapter 3. Apply to reduce the irritation of minor insect bites.

CONSIDERATIONS

Black cohosh is a powerful herb. It should not be taken if the possibility of pregnancy exists or if the patient has any type of chronic disease. Large doses of this herb can cause symptoms of poisoning. It is very beneficial so don't be afraid of it. Do remember not to take it for more than three days in a row.

Burdock *(Arctium lappa)*

Burdock is a valuable blood purifier and immune system stimulant with the potential to aid liver and gallblader function. It settles an upset stomach and stimulates the production of digestive juices. Burdock has been used to relieve gout since medieval times. When used externally as a wash, burdock is beneficial for skin conditions, including eczema, psoriasis, and canker sores. It also soothes itchy, irritated hemorrhoids.

DESCRIPTION AND PARTS USED

Burdock is often mistaken for a weed. This tall plant reaches a height of three to four feet and has coarse broad leaves and prickly burs that fasten themselves to the clothing of any passerby. Being a biennial, burdock flowers during its second year of growth. The valuable parts of this unattractive herb are the root and seeds.

HISTORICAL NOTES

Although burdock is native to Europe and was widely used in the Old World, it never made it into any of the pharmacopoeias of the times. However, it was a favorite of many of the master herbalists, including Parkinson and Culpeper. John Parkinson praised it as a remedy for poisonous bites, including that of the mad dog. Culpeper said the leaves were good for old lesions and sores, being "cooling and moderately drying." The leaves were often used in poultices. The colonists brought burdock with them to the New World and introduced this herb to the Native Americans.

SCIENTIFIC FINDINGS

Burdock contains biotin, copper, iron, manganese, zinc, volatile oils, sulfur, tannins, three B vitamins, and vitamin E.

TRADITIONAL USE

Internal. Prepare a decoction of burdock root in accordance with the general instructions given in Chapter 3. To help purify the blood in all cases of illness, especially when toxicity exists, take one to three cups of tea daily.

External. Prepare a strong decoction according to the directions given in Chapter 3. Apply to the affected area as needed.

CONSIDERATIONS

Be aware that when taken internally, burdock can interfere with iron absorption.

Calendula *(Calendula officinalis)*

Calendula is a noted febrifuge, but it does a lot more than break fevers. Calendula soothes stomach ulcers, relieves menstrual cramps, softens varicose veins, and fights eruptive skin diseases, including herpes zoster (shingles). Externally applied, the cooled tea soothes burns and promotes healing of open wounds. When used as eardrops, it reduces the pain and discomfort of an earache.

DESCRIPTION AND PARTS USED

Calendula is simply the familiar marigold in formal dress. The golden-red-orange flowers of the marigold are pleasing to the eye.

Because the plant grows compactly and hugs the ground, marigold is a very colorful and an extremely popular border plant that has been enjoyed both for its beauty and its healing qualities for centuries.

The flower petals hold the medicinal properties. Tiny petals must be plucked from the flower's head one by one, a laborious task, and dried without touching one another. The flower head is discarded.

HISTORICAL NOTES

The ancient Romans are responsible for the Latin name of this plant, which refers to the fact that calendula blooms on the day of the new moon, which was the first day of the month—*calends*—in the Roman calendar. The more familiar name originated in medieval England from the Anglo Saxon legend that described the Virgin Mary as wearing golden blossoms in her hair. The poets of the period dubbed this herb "Mary Gowles" and "Mary Golde," which was transformed over time into "marigold," the name by which we know calendula today.

SCIENTIFIC FINDINGS

Chinese studies praise calendula as a remedy for hemorrhoids. When taken internally, it prevents suppuration (weeping pus); applied externally, it relieves itching, soothes tender tissue, and relieves pain. Other research validates the old belief in calendula as a treatment for chronic ulcers.

TRADITIONAL USE

Internal. Brew a healing tea by steeping 1 heaping tablespoon (1/2 ounce or 12 grams) of dried calendula in 1 cup of freshly boiled water for 3 minutes. Take 1 cup of tea daily. (For more information on brewing tea, see Chapter 3.)

External. Calendula oil is available commercially in the form of eardrops and liquid extract. Both are useful to have on hand for quick relief of an earache or to treat cuts, scrapes, and small wounds.

Do not use calendula oil on a burn. Anything greasy or oily

holds in the heat and can actually move the burn deeper into the dermis. To soothe minor burns, simply apply cooled tea to the affected area.

Try rubbing a fresh marigold flower on a wasp or bee sting. You'll be surprised at how quickly the pain and swelling disappear.

CONSIDERATIONS

Marigold blossoms have been tossed into salads, soups, and stews for centuries. This herb is remarkably free of any toxic effects.

Capsicum

See Cayenne.

Cascara Sagrada
(Rhamnus purshiana)

Cascara is a champion colon cleanser and excellent laxative. It's considered helpful against liver disorders, gallstones, leukemia, colitis, and diverticulosis. Cascara is also an old-time vermifuge valuable for expelling intestinal parasites.

DESCRIPTION AND PARTS USED

Cascara sagrada is a bush (not a tree). This plant is native to California, although it has been found growing wild from northern Idaho west to the Pacific Ocean. The bark, which contains the medicinal properties, is collected from the young trunk and moderately-sized branches. The action of the bark becomes milder and less emetic once it has been dried. Dried bark that has been stored for three years is considered best for pharmaceutical purposes.

HISTORICAL NOTES

This native American plant was named cascara sagrada, or sacred bark, by the Spanish missionaries who learned of its value from the Native Americans they were attempting to convert. The bark of the cascara sagrada bush has been used for centuries as a powerful purge or gentle overnight laxative, depending on how densely it is concentrated in the brewing.

In the 1930s, an over-the-counter laxative named Fletcher's Castoria was a staple in every medicine cabinet. Its main ingredient was cascara bark.

SCIENTIFIC FINDINGS

Cascara sagrada acts principally on the large intestine to stimulate peristalsis. One of the advantages of this herb is that it has a toning action on the bowels. It is considered mild enough for the ill, the elderly, and the very young. The herb may be used in cases of chronic constipation without fear as the quantity taken needn't be increased the second and third time for it to work.

TRADITIONAL USE

Internal. Diluting 5 to 15 drops of tincture in a cup of water or tea is the usual method for taking advantage of cascara's laxative properties. However, a healing cup of cascara sagrada tea will overcome constipation overnight and tone up the bowels at the same time. Prepare the tea using 1 rounded teaspoon (1/6 ounce or 4 grams) of herb per cup. (For more information on brewing teas, see Chapter 3.)

CONSIDERATIONS

Bark from the common "purging" buckthorn, *Rhamnus cathartica*, can be mistaken for its more gentle cousin, *Rhamnus sagrada*. Buckthorn bark must be seasoned and aged carefully to inhibit its cathartic power. Even then, it is so violent in action that it can be dangerous. Before you brew, make sure you have the "sacred bark," not the "purging buckthorn." Be aware, too, that an excessive dose of cascara sagrada can cause severe cramps and diarrhea.

Be guided by the box as to the quantity of the herb to use when brewing a healing tea.

Cayenne
(*Capsicum frutescens* and *C. anuum*)

Capsicum, more familiarly known as cayenne pepper, potentiates all other herbs. This champion blood cleanser improves circulation, benefits the kidneys, lungs, spleen, pancreas, heart, and stomach. Cayenne has been used as a digestive aid and is one of the herbalist's specifics against nausea. With its anti-inflammatory properties, it is helpful in rheumatism, arthritis, and migraines. Cayenne even quickly relieves common cold symptoms.

Externally, cayenne has been used to good effect in ointments and salves for centuries. As a rubefacient, it produces penetrating heat to bring relief to aching muscles and painful joints.

DESCRIPTION AND PARTS USED

The Capsicum family includes cayenne peppers, red and green chillies, paprika, and bell peppers. Hot peppers, including cayenne, put forth small and slender fruits. The heat and medicinal properties are housed in the seeds.

HISTORICAL NOTES

Historically, cayenne is considered an excellent digestive aid because it stimulates the production of gastric juices, improves metabolism, and relieves gas. An old herbal suggests that when cayenne is rubbed into the scalp, it causes bald spots to sprout hair.

SCIENTIFIC FINDINGS

Peppers in general are rich in bioflavonoids and are considered very nutritious. The stimulating effect of cayenne comes from the hot, stinging sensation the muncher experiences upon biting into the hot pepper. According to researchers at UCLA, the sting and burning of the mucous membranes of the mouth trigger the release of endorphins, the brain chemicals that relieve pain and cause a mild euphoria. It has also been reported that capsicum is a neurotransmitter and, as such, is very effective against pain. Studies indicate that cayenne has been used successfully against "cluster" type migraines. Because it is a vasodilator, capsicum has also been used in the treatment of Raynaud's phenomenon. Of even more interest, a study published in the *Journal of Bioscience* in 1987 reported that lab animals fed a diet high in cayenne experienced a significant reduction in "bad" cholesterol.

TRADITIONAL USE

Internal. Prepare a healing tea using 1 rounded teaspoon of herb per cup. (For more information on brewing teas, see Chapter 3.) Take 1 to 3 cups daily for 3 days only. Do not use cayenne on a continuing basis. To take advantage of its catalytic action, add a quarter cup of cayenne tea to any other healing tea.

External. As an ingredient in ointments, liniments, and salves, cayenne warms deep down to help relieve the pain and stiffness of arthritic joints or overused muscles.

CONSIDERATIONS

Treat cayenne with great respect. It should not be used by anyone with a hiatus hernia or any gastrointestinal problems; it's just too strong for internal membranes that are already irritated. High doses taken internally can cause gastroenteritis and kidney damage.

You should know that this hot herb can now be purchased according to the number of heat units the preparation contains. For example, 30,000 to 40,000 heat units is considered mild, while 90,000 heat units is mighty hot. Consult your herbalist or staff in your health-food store for more information.

Don't use an ointment that contains cayenne on broken skin (or hemmorrhoids). Although it warms and soothes, prolonged use of cayenne can irritate the skin. Use with care.

Chamomile
(*Anthemis nobilis*
and *Matricaria chamomilla*)

Chamomile has been used for centuries as a calmative. It brews into a soothing nerve tonic, and insomniacs find it invaluable. A cup of chamomile tea before bed is said to prevent nightmares.

Chamomile stimulates a flagging appetite, improves digestion, encourages the bladder, relieves colitis, diverticulosis, and hemorrhoids. Chamomile is even beneficial in the treatment of rheumatism, arthritis, headaches, muscle cramps, and pain.

Chamomile tea has been used with some success against the delirium tremens sometimes suffered by alcoholics.

DESCRIPTION AND PARTS USED

It may suprise you to learn that there are two varieties of chamomile. For centuries, herbalists have argued over which variety—the Roman *Anthemis nobilis* or the German *Matricaria chamomilla*—is the most powerful medicinal. Don't worry about it. Their properties are nearly identical and certainly interchangeable. Both chamomiles have feathery foliage and daisylike flowers.

It always comes as a surprise to the uninitiated to discover that chamomile has a faint but distinctly applelike fragrance. Actually, its name is a direct reference to this fragrance. "Chamomile" is drawn from the ancient Greek for "on the ground"—*kamai*—and for "apple"—*melon*. The active constituents of chamomile are found in the flowers.

HISTORICAL NOTES

The ancient Egyptians held chamomile in such high esteem that it was dedicated to their highest god. An old herbal tells us, "Thys herbe was consecrated by the wyse men of Egypt unto the Sonne and was rekened to be the only remedy of all agues."

Dioscorides and Pliny recommended chamomile as a cure for headaches and all illnesses attacking the liver, kidneys, and bladder. Famous English herbalist Culpeper called chamomile "a hateful weed," but praised its medicinal qualities with these words, "It possess virtues that may recompense all the damage it can do among the corn. For those who have cold and weak stomachs, scarcely anything equals the Chamomiles. They are best taken by way of infusion, like tea."

SCIENTIFIC FINDINGS

Chamomile is recognized in Europe, especially in France and Spain, by many members of the orthodox medical profession who routinely prescribe the tea. It contains traces of vitamin A, a high level of calcium and magnesium, potassium, iron, manganese and zinc.

TRADITIONAL USE

Internal. Chamomile tea is brewed by steeping 1 tablespoon (1/2 ounce or 13 grams) of the dried flowers in an 8-ounce cup of freshly boiled water for 5 minutes. (For more information on brewing tea, see Chapter 3.)

External. A chamomile poultice is wonderfully soothing to sore muscles and painful joints; it helps reduce swelling. For directions on preparing a poultice, please refer to Chapter 3.

A chamomile wash or cup of brewed tea has been used for centuries as a hair rinse. Old herbals say it brightens and lightens blonde hair.

CONSIDERATIONS

Don't use chamomile if you are allergic to ragweed or subject to seasonal allergies. Although chamomile is considered mild and gentle, don't use it continuously over a long period of time. It is best taken as a healing tea for occasional use only.

Comfrey *(Symphytum officinale)*

Because comfrey may cause liver damage, the FDA no longer permits it to be sold for internal use. However, this herb is used with appropriate caution by knowledgeable herbalists. If you have some dried comfrey in your store of herbs, please pay attention to the warning given under Considerations below.

Historically, comfrey was considered a healing and soothing blood purifier used for strengthening the lungs, stomach, kidneys, and bowels. It is a demulcent and expectorant, traditionally used to treat asthma, coughs, and congestion. The leaves have been used to treat cramps, diarrhea, hemorrhage, ulcers, and tuberculosis.

Both internally and externally, this herb is considered to be a powerful and speedy healer of fractures and bone breaks of all kinds. When used topically, comfrey root fights inflammation, brings down swelling, helps heal wounds, burns, breaks, fractures, and bruises, and relieves pain.

DESCRIPTION AND PARTS USED

Comfrey tends to grow in large clumps and can reach a height of nearly three feet. It thrives in full sun, but does well in partial shade. This herb has large, fuzzy, dark-green leaves that are rough and pointed at the ends. Comfrey puts forth creamy yellow or purplish-blue flowers on stems that curve inward like a scorpion's tail. The plant likes moisture and makes a handsome addition to any garden. The medicinal properties are found in the leaves and roots.

HISTORICAL NOTES

Comfrey has a long and rich history. No herb garden or apothecary shop of the past was considered well-stocked without it. The herb's common name comes from a slurred corruption of the Latin term *con firma*, which refers to the old belief that it can firm and join broken bones. Its botanical name, *symphytum*, derives from the Greek *symphyto*, which means "to unite."

Comfrey has been used for centuries as a poultice or compress to treat wounds, ease swollen and inflammed joints, relieve the pain of bruises and burns, and help heal breaks. It is even said to eliminate the phantom pain that often occurs when a limb has been amputated.

Old-time healers were true believers. Master herbalist Culpeper wrote, "Comfrey is said to be so powerful to consolidate and knit together, if it be boyled with disservered pieces of flesh in a pot, it will join them together." He went on to say, "The Great Comfrey restrains spitting of blood. The roote boyled in water or wine and the decoction drank, heals inward hurts, bruises, woundes, and ulcers of the lungs and causes the catarrah and phlegm that oppresses to be easily spyt forth."

SCIENTIFIC FINDINGS

As far back as 1912, the *British Medical Journal* reported that the active properties of comfrey derived from the allantoin (a white crystalline substance) it contains. The article stated, in part, "Allantoin in aqueous solution has a powerful action in strengthening epithelial formation and is a valuable remedy for external ulcerations and ulcers of the stomach and duodenum."

Modern science has determined that the virtues of comfrey applied externally as a vulnerary, or wound-healer, come from the amount of allantoin it contains. Allantoin has proved so useful in treating wounds, burns, and ulcers that it is chemically synthesized.

TRADITIONAL USE

Internal. Comfrey should not be taken internally. If you insist that Culpeper was right and today's medical scientists are wrong, consult a knowledgeable herbalist who is aware of comfrey's potential for harm and who is well versed in the intricacies of herbal prescriptions.

External. If you are lucky enough to have comfrey growing outside your door, a quick and very effective poultice can be made by gathering a handful of the fresh leaves, scalding them quickly with boiling water, and applying them warm to the affected area. Use an overwrap to hold in the heat and keep the leaves in place.

Reapply as needed. (For instructions on other methods of preparing a compress or poultice, please see Chapter 3.)

CONSIDERATIONS

Comfrey is a powerful medicinal that may cause liver damage.

Damiana *(Turnera aphrodisiaca)*

As its botanical name suggests, damiana has been used for centuries to enhance sexual prowess and balance the hormones. Damiana is a unisex herb. It is traditionally considered valuable for increasing the sperm count in men, as well as for strengthening the ovaries of women.

This stimulating herb has also been used for nervousness, headache, chronic bed-wetting, weakness, and exhaustion. Damiana tea is considered particularly helpful in restoring energies lost to illness. It is reputed to revitalize the entire body.

DESCRIPTION AND PARTS USED

Damiana is a small plant that bears fragrant yellowish-white flowers. Its natural habitat is southern California, Texas, and Mexico. Damiana has been used "South of the Border" since ancient times, which explains why it is sometimes called "the Mexican aphrodisiac and tonic." The medicinal properties of damiana are stored in the leaves.

HISTORICAL NOTES

A manuscript inscribed in Latin in 1552 by a native Aztec doctor who was educated by Spanish missionaries describes many of the herbs used by the medicine men of the times, including damiana. As the colonists settled in the New World, Mexican medical knowledge inched its way into North American consciousness.

In Mexico today, herbal doctors run thriving practices in many of the larger cities, and most open-air markets have vendors of medicinal herbs. In spite of four centuries of European medical practice, the population still depends on local plants.

Experience shows that damiana tea really can be considered a type of "love potion." Taking the tea is said to cause the body to increase production of those pheromones (secretions that influence patterns of behavior) that attract the opposite sex. The effects of the tea are not immediate; they are cumulative. Before looking for those love-struck gazes from the one you wish to attract, you'll need to drink one cup a day of this stimulating tea for about a week.

SCIENTIFIC FINDINGS

Damiana is classified in the Mexican pharmacopoeia as an aphrodisiac, tonic, and diuretic. Scientists have accepted it as a reliable remedy in cases of sexual impotence, especially when the condition is caused by overindulgence leading to exhaustion.

Authoritative medical herbalists agree. In *Potter's Cyclopaedia of Botanical Drugs and Preparations*, the author says, "Damiana is very largly prescribed on account of its aphrodisiac qualities; there is no doubt that it has a very great and generally beneficial action on the reproductive system. It also acts as a tonic to the nervous system."

TRADITIONAL USE

Internal. Damiana tea is prepared with one teaspoon (1/6 ounce or 4 grams) of dried leaves to one cup of freshly boiled water. Cover, steep for five minutes, and drink upon rising, before eating. (For more information on brewing teas, see Chapter 3.)

CONSIDERATIONS

Damiana interferes with iron absorption and should be used only on an occasional basis.

Dandelion *(Taraxacum officinale)*

Dandelion is an effective blood and liver purifier; it increases the production of bile, aids digestion, and encourages the free flow of urine. It improves the functioning of the pancreas, spleen, liver, bladder, and kidneys. Dandelion is helpful against anemia, gout, hypoglycemia, rheumatism, jaundice, cirrhosis, hepatitis, cramps, and constipation. This powerful herb reduces levels of serum cholesterol and uric acid, and may even help prevent breast cancer.

Fresh young dandelion greens are a spring treat in many households. The bitter greens, often dressed with a dollop of vinegar, steam to tender, nutrient-rich perfection.

DESCRIPTION AND PARTS USED

The dandelion grows anywhere. Many people consider it a weed and dig it up furiously when the golden heads spoil the green of a well-tended lawn. Dandelions have thick, long tap roots, dark on the outside and white within. The toothed leaves rise directly from the root and form a rosette around the radius of the plant. Each stem bears one of the familiar bright yellow blossoms. The roots and leaves are medicinal storehouses.

HISTORICAL NOTES

The French called dandelion *dent de leon*; its original Latin name was *Dens leonis*, and the Greeks named it *Leontodon*. As you probably know, all these phrases translate into "tooth of the lion." The reference is to the deep, jagged "teeth" of the dandelion leaf, which suggested the fangs of the King of Beasts to those who named this herb and appreciated its powerful medicinal properties.

SCIENTIFIC FINDINGS

The dandelion is a storehouse of nutrients, including vitamins, minerals, and trace elements. It contains vitamins A, B-complex, C, and E, biotin, calcium, choline, inositol, iron, linolenic acid, magnesium, niacin, PABA, phosphorus, zinc, potash, proteins, resins, and sulfur. Dandelion, which stimulates metabolism by providing acids that are necessary for good digestion, has been shown to be helpful to stressed intestines.

TRADITIONAL USE

Internal. Dandelion tea is wonderfully healing. Just pour a cupful of freshly boiled water over 1 to 2 teaspoons (1/6 to 1/3 ounce or 4 to 8 grams) of the herb. Let the tea brew for 10 minutes before straining. (For more information on brewing tea, see Chapter 3.) For the full benefit of dandelion's whole-body tonic effects, drink 1 cupful in the morning and another in the evening for 4 to 8 weeks.

CONSIDERATIONS

In spite of all the power dandelion tea exerts, this natural medicinal is completely free of any toxic side effects.

Dong Quai *(Angelica sinensis)*

Although dong quai stimulates both ovarian and testicular hormones, it is known in Asia as the "female ginseng." It is primarily used to treat a host of female problems, especially those connected to the menses. Of all the Chinese medicinal plants, this herb is the most beneficial as treatment for cramps, PMS, irregular menstruation, hot flashes and other menopausal complaints; it even overcomes vaginal dryness.

Dong quai has a calming effect on the central nervous system, helps strengthen internal body organs, and increases circulation. This herb is historically considered the whole-body tea for women.

DESCRIPTION AND PARTS USED

This sweet and pungent herb is native to the Far East. Leafy foliage grows high up on rather spindly stems. The beneficial medicinal properties of dong quai are found in the stubby, whitish-gray roots of the plant. The roots, which have a pungent and distinctive odor, must be stored in a dry place so they don't soften and spoil.

HISTORICAL NOTES

Dong quai has been used in China for many thousands of years. According to Chinese medical lore, maintaining the youthful freshness of the female organs with nourishing dong quai tea delays the symptoms of old age in women. Because it strengthens female sexual organs and rejuvenates hormonal systems, dong quai is known as the "longevity herb" for women.

SCIENTIFIC FINDINGS

Dong quai contains essential oils, alcohols, carotene, sucrose, cadinene, carvacrol, isosafrol, safrol, and sesquiterpenes, plus vitamins A, B_{12}, and E. As a result of many studies, vitamin E has gained the reputation of being the "sex" and "longevity" vitamin.

TRADITIONAL USE

Internal. The Chinese method of using dong quai results in a very potent and nourishing broth. Here's the old method: Put four cups of pure water in an enamelware cooking pot. (The instructions caution specifically against using aluminum and say even stainless steel should not be used.) Put a few pieces of lean raw chicken or beef into the pot. Add one small dong quai root or half of a large root. Simmer the broth slowly for several hours or until the liquid is reduced by half. Strain and drink warm. Because of its power, a cup of this broth is taken just twice a month. It is taken without fail by those women who wish to maintain a youthful freshness.

If you prefer to brew a cup of dong quai tea for occasional use, you will need to brew a decoction (see Chapter 3 for instructions).

CONSIDERATIONS

Because it stimulates uterine contractions, dong quai should not be used during menstration (especially if the flow is heavy) or during pregnancy.

Echinacea *(Echinacea angustifolia)*

Echinacea, pronounced ek-ah-nay-sha, is helpful to the lymphatic system and is a powerful immune system stimulant. It fights viral and bacterial infections and has anti-inflammatory properties. Echinacea is useful in cases of colic, colds, flu, and infections of all kinds. A cup of echinacea tea should be drunk whenever the body is under attack.

Externally applied, echinacea fights infection, reduces inflammation, and promotes healing. It is useful against many skin conditions.

DESCRIPTION AND PARTS USED

Echinacea is native to the North American midwest. It typically grows from two to three feet high, puts forth several stems per clump, and has thick, hairy leaves that are anywhere from three to eight inches long. This perennial herb usually has one large, light purple flower per stem. The flowers appear during the second year of growth. The medicinal properties of echinacea are stored in the root.

HISTORICAL NOTES

Native Americans were using this medicinal long before the colonists arrived. The Sioux used echinacea for snakebite; the tribes of Nebraska used it as both a pain reliever and antiseptic. Chewing the root quickly healed a sore throat, and toothaches were treated by applying a piece of root directly on the affected tooth.

By the latter part of the nineteenth century, this herb was in common use as a blood purifier. Back then, echinacea tea was the doctor's treatment of choice for, in the words of an old American herbal, "bad blood with a tendency to sepsis and malignancy." As word of its effectiveness spread, echinacea became a favorite of European healers as well. Echinacea was one of the Shaker's most successful exports.

SCIENTIFIC FINDINGS

The immune-enhancing properties of echinacea have been documented in many studies. It has been shown to stimulate the production of white blood cells, the "soldiers" of the immune system, and to deactivate the enzyme hyaluronidase. Without this enzyme, invading organisms are less able to permeate tissues. The *Journal of Medical Chemistry* published a study in 1972 showing that an extract of echinacea slowed down the growth of tumors in lab animals. In 1977, *Planta Medica* published findings that an extract of echinacea destroyed herpes and influenza viruses in a test tube. Several sources have reported that the topical application of echinacea works against psoriasis, eczema, and the candida fungus.

TRADITIONAL USE

Internal. To prepare a healing tea using dried or powdered echinacea, use 1 to 2 teaspoons (1/6 to 1/3 ounce or 4 to 8 grams) of the herb per cup of freshly boiled pure water. (For more information on brewing tea, see Chapter 3.) If using a piece of the whole root, prepare a decoction (see Chapter 3) instead. To give the immune system a boost, take 1 cup of tea 3 times daily as a general stimulant.

External. Echinacea can promote healing and fight infection in many skin diseases and is helpful for cuts, sores, and minor burns. Even wounds and stubborn sores that refuse to close and heal will benefit from this traditional Native American remedy. To use, prepare a tea or strong wash following the directions given in Chapter 3.

CONSIDERATIONS

Echinacea is regarded as an extremely safe herb with virtually no reported instances of toxicity. When shopping for this herb, select a preparation that has been freeze-dried. The experts say that some of echinacea's active compounds can be lost if the herb is prepared in an alcohol-based tincture.

Ephedra *(Ephedra sinica)*

See **Mahuang.**

Essiac

See inset on page 129.

Eyebright *(Euphrasia officinalis)*

As its name suggests, eyebright is the herbalist's treatment of choice for all eye disorders. Taken internally, it is traditionally believed capable of maintaining healthy eyes and good vision. Externally, eyebright is used as a mild eyewash with antiseptic properties. It is valuable for preventing the constant and annoying watering of weak eyes and helps relieve eyes that are particularly sensitive to light. Eyebright can quickly eliminate discomfort arising from conjunctivitis, blepharitis, eyestrain, inflammation, sties, or minor irritation.

DESCRIPTION AND PARTS USED

Eyebright is familiar in Britain, but is seldom grown on this side of the Atlantic. Because the herb has a symbiotic relationship with grass, the British people think of it as a weed. Eyebright roots send out tiny feelers that attach themselves to the roots of grasses and draw nourishment from them. This elegant little annual attains a modest height of two to eight inches. It puts forth deeply cut leaves and becomes covered with many small white or purple flowers that are speckled with yellow. Except for those pesky roots, the entire herb is useful.

HISTORICAL NOTES

Eyebright has been used since the Middle Ages as an eyewash and tonic tea for the eyes. In days gone by, delicate children who were especially prone to weak and watering eyes and runny noses were dosed with eyebright tea first thing in the morning and last thing at night. It is written that this cure is most efficacious if continued over a period of months.

SCIENTIFIC FINDINGS

Eyebright is extremely rich in the "eye vitamin"—vitamin A— and in vitamin C. It also contains moderate amounts of B complex, D, and traces of vitamin E, and offers iron and silicon, plus traces of iodine, copper, and zinc.

TRADITIONAL USE

Internal. If you wish to try easing your eyes from the inside-out, you can prepare a healing tea by using 1 rounded teaspoon (1/6 ounce or 4 grams) of eyebright to 1 cup of water. (For more information on brewing tea, see Chapter 3.)

External. For an eyebright eyewash, put 1 teaspoon of the herb in 1 cupful of water and bring to a boil. To make the tea more compatible with the normal saline in the eyes, add the tiniest smidgen of salt. Simmer for 2 minutes. Cool to body temperature.

An eyebright compress is wonderfully soothing to tired, irritated eyes. For directions on preparing a compress, please see Chapter 3.

CONSIDERATIONS

In centuries of use, eyebright has left behind no record of complaints.

Essiac—
Rene Caisse's Cancer Formula

Every few years, information about Essiac resurfaces when its history appears in articles or books. A nurse named Rene Caisse is credited with having created the formula, which she dubbed "Essiac," her last name spelled backwards.

Born in Bracebridge, Ontario, Canada, in 1888, Caisse was nursing an aged patient with a scarred breast in an Ontario hospital in 1922. The woman told Caisse that many years earlier she had been diagnosed with breast cancer and scheduled for a mastectomy. However, a Chippawa Indian neighbor offered her an herbal tea, which she took. Over time, the wonderful tea eliminated the cancer completely. Caisse asked for the herbal formula, which she herself later strengthened and subsequently used to cure her aunt of inoperable stomach cancer.

When Caisse treated other terminal cancer patients with Essiac tea and they began to show improvement, several Canadian physicians became interested. Two petitions ensued, one in 1926 and one in 1936, seeking approval from Ottawa's Department of Health and Welfare so that Caisse could dispense Essiac to cancer patients on a much larger scale. Both petitions were rejected. In 1938, a bill was submitted to the Canadian government in an effort to legalize Essiac as a cancer remedy for terminal patients. That bill failed to pass by just three votes. Nonetheless, Caisse continued to supply Essiac to those who needed it, and the success stories continued to mount.

In 1977, one year before her death, Caisse turned over the formula for Essiac to the Resperin Corporation of Ontario for the sum of $1.00. Her hope was that Resperin's board of directors would succeed in setting up trial studies of the formula that would result in the scientific and clinical documentation needed to market Essiac as a true drug. That still hasn't happened. Although Resperin made the formula available to interested physicians, many of the doctors who reported back to Resperin had negative results. Today, only word-of-mouth reports, a few articles, and a book or two keep alive Rene Caisse's dream of aiding cancer victims with Essiac.

Essiac is a combination tea consisting of four herbs: sheep's sorrel, burdock root, slippery elm bark, and turkey rhubarb root. Anecdotal evidence supplied by those who say they have eliminated cancer by taking Essiac tea is very persuasive. True double-blind studies of the formula are lacking, but the benefits of the individual plants used in the formula have long been praised.

Sheep's sorrel (Rumex acetosella), is a small perennial cousin of the common garden sorrel. This little plant grows abundantly in woodlands and shady places. The leaves, which hold the healing properties of the plant, are thin and delicate, brilliantly green above, faintly purple on their undersides. Sheep's sorrel is said to brew into a cooling, thirst-quenching tea with notable blood-purifying properties. This herb helps strengthen a weak stomach, can stimulate a convalescent's appetite, and is useful against nausea and vomiting.

Burdock (Arctium lappa), a burr-bearing biennial some call a weed, has large leaves and puts forth round heads of purple flowers. It reaches about three to four feet in height. The medicinal properties are housed in its inch-thick roots, which are typically about a foot in length, although they can be as long as the plant is tall. The highest quality root comes from the plant's first year of growth. Burdock root once appeared in American pharmacopoeias as a diuretic and diaphoretic. This mucilaginous herb is considered a champion blood purifier and good digestive aid. It has been found useful against coughs and sore throats.

Slippery elm (Ulmus fulva), is a small tree long valued for the medicinal properties of its inner bark. This variety of elm is indigenous to North America and Canada, where it grows abundantly. The bark is rough and flexible, with a reddish-yellow or reddish-brown outer covering. The inner bark shows striations along its full length. Herbalists say a tea brewed from slippery elm bark is both strengthening and healing, It is said to have emollient, expectorant, and diuretic properties. When made into a gruel, this herb has as much nutrition as oatmeal. It is considered a wholesome and sustaining food in its own right and is particularly suitable for infants and invalids.

Turkey rhubarb (Rheum palmatum), indigenous to China and Tibet, is much larger than the garden variety of rhubarb used in pies. It has a thick oval root that sends off long, tapering branches.

The root, which is the part used medicinally, is brown on the outside and a deep golden yellow on the inside. Turkey rhubarb root is credited with tonic and digestive properties. Although it is an effective purge, this herb has been used with notable success against dysentery. In a 1921 article in "Lancet," Dr. R. W. Burkitt wrote, "I know of no remedy in medicine that has such a magical effect. No one who has ever used rhubarb would dream of using anything else."

With the exception of burdock, which can interfere with iron absorption, the herbs contained in the Essiac formula carry no warnings when taken in moderation. Nonetheless, because there are many factors to be considered, anyone thinking of taking Esslac should read the very thorough and well-researched discussion of Essiac in "Options: The Alternative Cancer Therapy Book" by Richard Walters. Before you pin your hopes on this remedy, please consult that book, which was published in 1993. (If you don't find this work locally, the name and address of the publisher are listed in Sources of Information.)

In its Summer 1991 issue, "The Canadian Journal of Herbalism" published an article by Sheila Snow entitled, "Old Ontario Remedies: 1922: Rene Caisse: Essiac." The formula that appeared in that article is based on the Dr. Gary L. Glum's formula, which appears below.

Essiac Formula

Equipment:
4-gallon stainless steel pot, with lid
3-gallon stainless steel pot, with lid
Stainless steel fine-mesh double strainer
Stainless steel funnel
Stainless steel spatula
12 or more 16-ounce sterilized amber glass bottles
with airtight caps
Measuring cup
Kitchen scale with ounce measurements

Ingredients:
6 1/2 cups burdock root, cut
16 ounces sheep sorrel herb, powdered
1 ounce turkey rhubarb root, powdered
4 ounces slippery elm bark, powdered
2 gallons sodium-free distilled water

1. Mix dry ingredients thoroughly. (Place herbs in plastic bag and shake vigorously.)

2. Bring water to a rolling boil in 4-gallon pot with lid on (approximately 30 minutes at sea level.)

3. Stir in 1 cup of dry ingredients. (Store remainder of herbs in a cool dark place; herbs are light sensitive.) Replace lid and continue boiling for 10 minutes.

4. Turn off stove. Scrape down sides of pot with spatula. Stir thoroughly. Replace lid.

5. Let pot stand, covered, for 12 hours. Turn stove to highest setting and heat pot almost to boiling, approximately 20 minutes. (Do not let mixture boil.)

6. Turn off stove. Strain liquid into 3-gallon pot. Clean 4-gallon pot and strainer. Strain liquid back into 4-gallon pot.

7. Use funnel to pour hot liquid immediately into sterilized bottles, taking care to tighten caps. Allow bottles to cool; then tighten caps again.

8. Refrigerate; the formula contains no preservative agents. If mold develops in bottle, discard immediately.

Caution: All bottles and caps must be sterilized after use if you plan to re-use them for this formula. You may use a 3 percent solution of food grade hydrogen perioxide in water. To make this solution, mix 1 ounce of 35 percent food grade hydrogen peroxide with 11 ounces of sodium-free distilled water. Let soak for 5 minutes. Rinse and dry. (If food grade hydrogen peroxide is not available, use 1/2 teaspoon of Clorox in 1 gallon of distilled water.)

Directions for use as a preventive
Shake the bottle. Take 4 tablespoons at bedtime on an empty stomach (at least two hours after eating). Formula may be taken cold from the bottle or heated. Do not microwave.

Directions for use by cancer and AIDS patients
Take 4 tablespoons in the morning. You may eat 5 minutes after taking the formula. Take 4 tablespoons again at bedtime, at least 2 hours after eating. If you have stomach cancer, the formula must be diluted with an equal amount of sodium-free distilled water before taking.

Feverfew *(Chrysanthemum parthenium)*

Feverfew is extremely helpful against headaches, even migraines, and is of great benefit to those who suffer from arthritis. This herb relieves fever and stimulates weak appetite in a convalescent. It helps ease symptoms of the common cold by increasing the fluidity of mucus caught in the lungs and bronchial tubes. Although not as powerful as dong quai (see page 123), feverfew stimulates uterine contractions, relieves cramps, and brings on menstrual flow.

DESCRIPTION AND PARTS USED

This hardy herb attains a height of two to three feet. The slender trunk of each stem branches out into several stems that bear alternating toothed leaves of a golden-green hue. The noted English herbalist Gerard described what he called "Featherfew" with these words: "It be tender, diversely torne and jagged, and nickt on the edges." Feverfew flowers are small and similar to daisies in appearance, with yellow centers and white, rayed petals.

The entire plant is filled with beneficial elements. Appreciated for its medicinal properties, feverfew is often cultivated throughout Europe and the United States.

HISTORICAL NOTES

The name feverfew is almost certainly a corruption of "febrifuge."
As such, the name is a nod of acknowledgement to but one of this
herb's many uses.

Culpeper, another of England's master herbalists, penned
these words on feverfew centuries ago:

> The powder of the herb taken in wine, purges both choler and
> phllegm, and is available for those that are short-winded, and
> those troubled with melancholy and heaviness or sadness of
> spirits. It is very effectual for all pains in the head, the herb
> being bruised and applied to the crown, as also for the vertigo,
> a running or swimming in the head.

Another herbal says, "In the worst headache, this herb ex-
ceeds whatever else be known. This herb is very effectual against
all pains in the head." I suppose a toothache qualifies as a "pain
in the head"; Cotton Mather, a New England colonist of note,
recommended feverfew be sprinkled with rum and applied hot to
relieve the pain of toothache.

To insure the most potent medicinal qualities when harvesting
home-grown feverfew, consider these instructions from an old
herbal: "Feverfew be most efficacious against ague and fever if the
herb be gathered with the left hand while speaking the name of
the patient aloud; but nary a glance behind shall ye dast."

SCIENTIFIC FINDINGS

Somewhere along the way, feverfew fell out of favor and was
almost forgotten until 1978 when the tale of a British woman who
cured her migraines with feverfew hit the London papers. The
story was so convincing that medical researchers became interested. It took a while for the results to come in, but the upshot
was a serious report in the British medical journal *Lancet* in 1985.
The report states that feverfew inhibits the release of two inflammatory substances thought to be the culprits in severe migraines
and the painful swollen joints characteristic of rheumatoid arthritis.

In 1988, *Lancet* stated the obvious by confirming what natural healers have known for centuries: Feverfew can prevent migraine headaches and/or lessen their severity, and is of great aid to the victims of arthritis. *Lancet* also reported this noteworthy item: Feverfew achieved much greater inhibition of the inflammatory agents responsible for so much pain in migraines and arthritis and was more effective than aspirin and other NSAIDs (nonsteroidal anti-inflammatory drugs).

TRADITIONAL USE

Internal. The standard use of feverfew is 3 cups of healing tea daily. Use 1 heaping teaspoon (1/6 ounce or 4 grams) of the herb to 1 cup of freshly boiled water. Cover and steep for 3 minutes. Strain and sip hot. (For more information on brewing tea, see Chapter 3.)

CONSIDERATIONS

The anti-inflammatory effects of feverfew are cumulative. Don't expect one cup of feverfew tea to banish arthritis and migraines forever. Herbs don't work like drugs. If you are faithful, you can expect good results within two weeks to a month and excellent results by the end of two months.

Here's a bit of encouragement and a warning all in one. During a six-month study of feverfew in the London Migraine Clinic, two patients who had successfully been treating their migraines with feverfew tea participated in the trial and were given a placebo or inert substance. As the effects of the feverfew in their systems wore off, their migraines came back full force. The two women left the study, went home to their feverfew tea, suffered while waiting for the herb to do its work, and finally sighed with relief when their migraines went back into remission.

Feverfew has been used for centuries with no ill effects. However, Cotton Mather's recommendation aside, chewing the leaves for toothache can cause canker sores. Some sensitive persons may develop a rash if the fresh herb touches their skin before it has been dried.

Garlic *(Allium sativum)*

Garlic is a very useful broad-spectrum whole-body detoxicant that fights infection of all types. This ancient herb supports the immune system and has antibiotic, antifungal, antimicrobial, and even antiviral properties. It strengthens blood vessels, helps regulate blood pressure, and reduces cholesterol. Garlic is useful in the treatment of arteriosclerosis, asthma, arthritis, cancer, circulatory problems, digestive disorders, liver disease, and ulcers. It combats sinusitis, helps relieve cold and flu symptoms, and may even help you sleep.

DESCRIPTION AND PARTS USED

Garlic is so well-known it needs no introduction. This perennial plant, a member of the lily family, is cultivated around the world. The cloves tucked inside the bulb hold the active elements. Garlic is appreciated both for its medicinal qualities and for the intense and distinctive flavor it brings to food.

HISTORICAL NOTES

The Chinese have known and used garlic for centuries, as have the peoples of the middle East. A four-thousand-year-old Chinese scroll entitled the *Calendar of the Hsai* mentions garlic. It was on the Babylonian menu in 3,000 B.C., and ancient Talmudic law stipulates garlic be used in certain dishes and on certain occasions. An Egyptian papyrus dating back to 1550 B.C. mentions garlic as an effective remedy against common ailments, including hypertension, tumors, bites, and worms.

Garlic has been around so long, almost every record of natural medicinals mentions it. In 1609, Sir John Harrington wrote the following in *The Englishman's Doctor*:

> Garlic then have the power to save from death
> Bear with it though it maketh unsavory breath,
> And scorn not garlic like some that think
> It only maketh men wink and drink and stink.

Although acknowledging garlic to be a theriacle—or cure-all—another old English herbal put it this way:

> . . . Garlick, Allium: thought a Charm against all Infection and Poyson (by which it has obtain'd the Name of the Country-man's Theriacle), we yet absolutely forbid it entrance into our Salleting, by reason of its intolerable Rankness, and which made it so detested of old that the eating of it was (as we read) part of the Punishment for such as had committed the horrid'st Crimes.

The written records of many civilizations speak of garlic, often called "stinkweed." The message is universal. It goes something like this: Garlic will heal many different ailments; the smell offends the nostrils.

SCIENTIFIC FINDINGS

The volatile oil in garlic is composed of several compounds that contain sulfur. These compounds are believed responsible for garlic's pharmacological actions. The following effects of garlic have been scientifically documented: It is antimicrobial, antibacterial, anticarcinogenic, antifungal, anthelmintic, anti-inflammatory, and antiviral. The heart-protective effects of garlic have also been scientifically established. Studies show garlic has a lipid-lowering effect; it decreases total serum cholesterol, while increasing HDL (high-density lipoproteins), the "good" cholesterol. In both animals and humans, garlic has been shown to decrease systolic blood pressure by twenty to thirty points and diastolic pressure by ten to twenty points.

Researchers testing garlic to lower cholesterol noticed that the subjects reported feeling less anxious, agitated, and irritable. It was subsequently determined that garlic affects the brain's release of serotonin, a chemical involved in regulating moods and behavior. When levels of serotonin in the brain are high, people tend to be calmer and less depressed.

TRADITIONAL USE

Internal. Garlic has long been taken for its medicinal properties. To reduce tension, one clove of garlic is crushed, left overnight in a glass of water, and drunk upon rising. In olden days, a

Garlic Syrup

Garlic does "brew" into a quite marvelous syrup. The effectiveness of this natural medicinal is so powerful, that it simply had to be included here in some form. Accordingly, here's a very old "receipt" for Garlic Syrup.

> *1 pound peeled and crushed garlic cloves*
> *apple cider vinegar*
> *pure water*
> *1 cup glycerine (available at pharmacies)*
> *1 cup honey*

1. *Put the peeled and crushed garlic cloves in a wide-mouthed 2-quart jar. Add equal parts of apple cider vinegar and pure water until the jar is 3/4 full. Cap the jar loosely and let the mixture stand in a warm place for 4 days. Shake the jar several times a day.*

2. *Add the glycerine. Shake to blend. Allow the mixture to stand in a warm place for 1 more day, shaking several times.*

3. *Strain the mixture through cheesecloth or muslin, squeezing to remove all the exhausted bits of garlic. Return the mixture to the jar.*

4. *Add the honey and stir until thoroughly mixed. Store the garlic syrup in a cool, dry place.*

Great-grandmother's directions

For coughs, colds, sore throats, bronchial congestion, high or low blood pressure, heart weakness, or nervous disorders, take 1 tablespoon of the syrup 3 times a day before meals.

decoction was used to treat worms and dropsy. Although I've never tried making garlic tea, if you want to sample such a concoction, simply use one small clove and follow the directions given in Chapter 3 for preparing a decoction.

External. Garlic oil is a time-honored folk remedy for earache. (See Chapter 3 for information on preparing an herbal oil.) A garlic juice douche is an old and very effective remedy for vaginal yeast infections. If you don't have a juicer, garlic juice can be purchased at health-food stores.

CONSIDERATIONS

Most people tolerate garlic comfortably, both inside and out. Some rare individuals may suffer an irritated digestive tract; even fewer may break out in a rash on contact with fresh garlic.

Ginger *(Zingiber officinales)*

This spicy delight is a specific for nausea, vomiting, motion sickness, gas, stomach cramps, and abdominal spasms. It is a good digestive aid, helps keep the colon clean, and fights colitis and diverticulosis. Because it helps reduce congestion and can ease a sore throat, ginger is a pleasant way to fight off colds and flu and clear the respiratory system. On the distaff side, ginger relieves morning sickness, eases menstrual cramps, and reduces hot flashes.

DESCRIPTION AND PARTS USED

Ginger is a low, spreading plant with heart-shaped leaves. It's very much at home in moist rich soil and likes partial shade. In early spring, it bears purplish-brown flowers. The medicinal properties reside in the root.

HISTORICAL NOTES

Dried ginger root has been used for thousands of years in Chinese medicine and in Chinese cookery. Wild ginger (*Asarum canadense*) once grew throughout our woodlands, but it's almost all gone now. Before the first explorers came to North America, Native Americans were using wild ginger to sweeten a sour stomach and fight nausea. American colonists discovered they liked the flavor ginger gave to hominy. Although it is not a preservative, most Europeans used ginger to cover up the taste and smell of tainted meat.

SCIENTIFIC FINDINGS

Ginger's legendary ability to improve digestion and relieve gastro-intestinal distress has been validated in recent experiments. In double-blind studies, ginger proved more effective at eliminating motion sickness than the over-the-counter drug Dramamine. Ginger reduced all the nasty symptoms associated with motion sickness, including dizziness, nausea, vomiting, cold sweats, and what sufferers call the "sick" headache that often signals an attack.

Pregnant mothers may rejoice to learn that research shows ginger eliminates morning sickness, even the form called hyperemesis gravidarum that can be severe enough to require hospitalization, without posing a danger to the unborn child. The effective dosage was 250 mg of powdered ginger root four times daily.

According to an article by Albert Leung, M.D., published in the *Journal of New Chinese Medicine*, the juice of fresh, crushed ginger root makes an excellent treatment for minor burns and skin inflammations.

TRADITIONAL USE

Internal. Ginger tea is very beneficial to the body. You can't steep this one; you need to brew a decoction. Grate 1 ounce (28 1/3 grams) of fresh or 1/2 ounce of dried ginger root. Simmer for 10 minutes in 1 pint of pure water. (For more information on preparing a decoction, see Chapter 3.) Sweetened with honey, ginger tea eases indigestion, cramps, and nausea. Add both honey and lemon, and this healing tea becomes a body-stimulating traditional cold, sore throat, and flu remedy.

External. For the relief of painful, swollen joints or sore, aching muscles, prepare a ginger fomentation or poultice. (See Chapter 3 for instructions.)

CONSIDERATIONS

Ginger can be used liberally by almost everyone.

Ginkgo *(Ginkgo biloba)*

Ginkgo powerfully stimulates the vast network of blood vessels that deliver blood and oxygen throughout the body. Because it even increases blood flow to the brain, it is one of the best natural medicinals for age-related disorders, including Alzheimer's disease, senility, and memory loss, as well as depression. Ginkgo has long been used to rev up a sluggish circulatory system, as well as to treat heart and kidney disorders. Gingko is even considered helpful against asthma and tinnitus (ringing in the ears).

DESCRIPTION AND PARTS USED

The ginkgo tree grows to a height of 100 to 125 feet and its trunk can be as large as 3 or 4 feet in diameter. Ginkgo trees can live as long as 1,000 years and have short, horizontal branches that put forth short shoots. Each shoot bears fan-shaped leaves, in which the medicinal properties are stored. This odd tree bears a nasty-smelling inedible fruit with a tasty almond-shaped inner seed. The seeds are edible and are sold in marketplaces all over Asia.

HISTORICAL NOTES

The ginkgo tree can be traced back more than 200 million years. Because it is the sole surviving member of the family *Ginkgoaceae*, it is sometimes referred to as a "living fossil." Although we tend to think of ginkgo as exclusive to the Chinese, it wasn't always so. Surprisingly, ginkgo once flourished in North America and Europe, but most gingko trees were destroyed during the Ice Age. The species survived only in China, where it is regarded as a sacred tree. Today, it is cultivated in the United States and valued only for its ornamental qualities.

Ginkgo's medicinal use can be traced back to a Chinese materia medica dated around 2800 B.C. The leaves have long been used in traditional Chinese medicine for their ability to "benefit the brain," the same properties for which we value them today.

SCIENTIFIC FINDINGS

In addition to improving blood supply to the brain, ginkgo also increases the rate at which information is transmitted at the nerve cell level, explaining why it is of such benefit in age-related disorders. In a double-blind study, the time of reaction of subjects performing a memory test improved significantly after *Ginkgo bilboa* extract (GBE) was administered. In another clinical study, the extract brought about a partial restoration of mental function in elderly patients. Here's the concluding statement to yet another study: "GBE medication has a positive effect in geriatric subjects with deterioration of mental performance and vigilance, and this effect is reflected at the behavioral level."

TRADITIONAL USE

Internal. In many clinical studies, a standardized extract of GBE was used at a dosage of 40 mg 3 times daily. A daily dose of 1 ounce (7 teaspoons or 28 1/3 grams) of a 1:5 tincture prepared from ginkgo leaf (readily available in health-food stores), is equivalent to the experimental dose.

All studies indicate that GBE should be taken consistently for at least 12 weeks in order to determine effectiveness. Although most subjects report benefits within 3 weeks, some may take longer to respond. In reviewing 20 studies involving almost 800 patients, it was reported that the longer the treatment continued, the more obvious and lasting the results. Even at the end of a year, improvements continued in those taking the extract.

CONSIDERATIONS

By all accounts, the long-term use of *Ginkgo biloba* is believed to be quite safe. No known serious side effects have been reported.

Ginseng, Chinese or Korean
(Panax ginseng),
Ginseng, Siberian
(Eleutherococcus senticosus),
Ginseng, American
(Panax quinquefolius)

The tonic effects of ginseng are legendary; it is—in fact and legend—an energizing whole-body tea. It is a noted strengthener of the immune system and helps against both mental and physical stress. Ginseng is considered particularly useful for rebuilding a weakened body and helping to speed recovery from illness. Ginseng is traditionally used to enhance sexual performance and improve sexual function. It stimulates the male sex glands and has proven successful against certain types of impotence. Ginseng provides measurable protection against radiation. Cancer patients find it softens the side effects of radiation treatment.

DESCRIPTION AND PARTS USED

The root is the repository of ginseng's medicinal elements. Chinese and Korean ginseng (*Panax ginseng*) is a small perennial plant widely cultivated for its taproot. The roots of the plant are white when dried; red when steamed. Old, wild, well-formed roots are the most valued; rootlets of the cultivated plants are considered the lowest grade. Roots between four and six years of age are the most potent.

Siberian ginseng (*Eleutherococcus senticosus*) is a small shrub that grows abundantly in Russia, Korea, China, and Japan north of latitude 38. Its distribution is much greater than that of *Panax ginseng*. The root is the most widely used medicinal part, but the leaves can also be of value.

American ginseng (*Panax quinquefolius*) is very similar to Chinese and Korean ginseng, although it is considered milder and less stimulating. Wisconsin-grown ginseng root is exported to the Orient where its gentleness is much appreciated. American ginseng is considered particularly suitable for convalescents.

HISTORICAL NOTES

Ginseng is one of the most honored and ancient of all medicinal herbs. Its recorded use in Chinese herbal medicine dates back more than 4,000 years. The Chinese value both *Panax* and *Eleuthero* and believe its regular use will increase longevity, improve general health, strengthen a weak appetite, and restore memory. Ginseng's value has been immortalized in the following lines from a very old Chinese parchment:

> *Ode to Wujia*
> How wonderful is Winzhang-grass, the Eleuthero-ginseng
> Dispensing in liquor for drinking,
> And decocting with burnet for daily using,
> It will keep your virgin face younger
> And prolong your life for ever and ever;
> Even a cartload of gold and jewels,
> Can not estimate your price of nature.

Native Americans used wild ginseng root to relieve nausea and vomiting. It was also much valued as a powerful addition to love potions. By the 1700s, American colonists knew and used this root. In the nineteenth century, a group of physicians known as the Eccletics, who rejected the growing trend toward manmade drugs prescribed ginseng as an aphrodisiac.

SCIENTIFIC FINDINGS

Serious research to determine if the properties attributed to ginseng are fact or fancy began in the 1950s. Many tests have confirmed the adaptogenic effects of ginseng. An adaptogen is a normalizing substance that increases resistance by virtue of a wide range of physical and chemical factors, no matter what the underlying cause of the problem may be. In other words, ginseng is a wonderful whole-body tonic tea, just as the ancients claimed.

Human studies to substantiate ginseng's legendary powers to enhance sexual function are in short supply. However, studies with animals have shown that ginseng promotes the growth of the testes and increases sperm formation in rabbits, accelerates the growth of the ovaries and stimulates ovulation in frogs, increases egg laying in hens, increases gonadal weight in both male and female rats, and increases sexual activity and mating behavior in male rats.

TRADITIONAL USE

Internal. The dosage of ginseng is directly tied to its ginsenoside content. Ginsenosides are the active components of all ginsengs. Of all ginsengs, the Korean and Chinese species test highest in these active components. If the tea contains a high concentration of ginsenosides and the other active components in ginseng, a lower dose will do the trick. The standard dose for a high-quality tea brewed from ginseng root is between 1 to 1 1/2 teaspoons (1/6 to 1/4 ounce or 4 to 6 grams) daily. To brew a decoction, necessary when dealing with a root, please see Chapter 3.

CONSIDERATIONS

In 1979, the *Journal of the American Medical Association (JAMA)* published an article entitled "Ginseng Abuse Syndrome" that listed the side effects of ginseng overuse as hypertension, euphoria, nervousness, insomnia, skin eruptions, and morning diarrhea. You should know that the commercial preparations *JAMA* reported on contained varying amounts of ginseng and were not subject to controlled analysis. Some preparations also contained additives and adulterants, a factor to consider. The article concluded with this sensible statement: "An important caveat is that these effects are neither uniformly negative nor uniformly predictable. Nevertheless, long-term use of large amounts of ginseng should be avoided. Even a panacea can cause problems if abused."

Studies performed with standardized extracts of ginseng have consistently demonstrated the absence of harmful side effects. Because you will be brewing your own healing tea, it is sensible to start slowly and monitor your body for any adverse reactions.

Goldenseal *(Hydrastis canadensis)*

Goldenseal enjoys a reputation as a cure-all, probably because it boosts immune function, and has anti-inflammatory, antibiotic, and antibacterial properties. This bitter herb is a good all-body purifier that aids the heart, lymphatic system, gastrointestinal tract, respiratory system, genitourinary tract, liver, spleen, pancreas, and colon. Goldenseal improves the action of sluggish glands and promotes hormonal harmony.

It is particularly useful as a healer of irritated mucous membranes throughout the body, which explains why goldenseal has a long tradition of use against colds, flu, glandular swelling, gum disease, and yeast infections.

DESCRIPTION AND PARTS USED

Goldenseal is a perennial herb that attains a modest height of about six inches. It bears a pair of five- to nine-lobed rounded leaves near the top of its single stem, which puts forth a single greenish-white flower. Goldenseal is native to North America and widely cultivated in Oregon and Washington for its medicinal qualities, which are stored in the roots and rhizomes.

HISTORICAL NOTES

The common name of this herb, goldenseal, refers to the rich golden stain the root leaves on everything it touches. Native Americans used the root to make an intense yellow dye as well as to derive medicinal benefits. A learned Native American healer in the nineteenth century wrote:

> The golden root is one of the Indian's favorite remedies; and medical men of the present age recognize it as one of the standard remedies for many pathological conditions or diseases of the human body. Too much cannot be said of this valuable agent, that has been veiled in darkness to the medical world for so long. I consider it one of the kings of diseases of the mucous membranes. It is unsurpassed by any known remedy.

The dried rhizome and root of goldenseal were first listed in the *United States Pharmacopoeia* in 1831. It was dropped in 1842, reinstated in 1863, and remained on the official list of drug plants until 1936. The popularity of goldenseal almost brought about its demise. Foragers were getting $1.50 per pound for goldenseal root at a time when most medicinal herbs were commanding only 2-5¢ per pound. Fortunately, commerical cultivation of this herb saved it from extinction. It brought the price down, too.

SCIENTIFIC FINDINGS

The medicinal value of goldenseal is believed to derive from its high content of berberine, an alkoloid constituent that has been widely studied. Research shows it has powerful antibiotic and immunostimulatory qualities. In controlled studies, berberine increased blood supply to the spleen, an organ responsible for filtering the blood and releasing specific compounds that potentiate immune function. Berberine activates macrophages, immune system cells that destroy bacteria, viruses, tumor cells, and other harmful foreign substances. Berberine's ability to inhibit the growth of the Candida organism, responsible for so many yeast infections, has also been documented. Beribine has often proven to be more effective against disease-producing organisms than many synthetic antibiotics currently being used.

TRADITIONAL PREPARATION

Internal. If you are using the dried root, brew a healing decoction using 1/2 to 1 teaspoon (1/12 to 1/6 ounce or 2 to 4 grams) of goldenseal root. (For more information on decoctions, see Chapter 3.) Take 1 cup of tea 3 times daily.

Goldenseal root is also available in powdered form. To use, add 1 teaspoon of goldenseal powder to 1 pint of hot water. Stir until the powder dissolves and let the tea stand until cool. Take 1 to 2 teaspoons 3 to 6 times daily.

External. A goldenseal douche can relieve yeast infections, such as Candida. Dissolve one tablespoon of powder in 1 quart of warm water. Let cool. Douche once every third day for up to 2 weeks.

Goldenseal tea is helpful in healing skin ailments, irritated gums, and canker sores. It offers both antiseptic and anti-inflammatory action when used as a wash. (For information on preparing washes, see Chapter 3).

CONSIDERATIONS

Do not use goldenseal for more than two weeks at a time. Because goldenseal can raise blood pressure, it should not be used by anyone with a history of—or potential for—high blood pressure. Do not use goldenseal during pregnancy.

Gotu Kola *(Centella asiatica)*

This medicinal herb of India, known as Brahmi in the Ayurvedic tradition, stimulates the central nervous system, rebuilds energy reserves, relieves high blood pressure, and helps the body defend against various toxins. Gotu kola is used to treat rheumatism, blood diseases, congestive heart failure, urinary tract infections, venereal diseases, hepatitis, and high blood pressure. It is a mild diuretic that can help shrink swollen membranes and aid in the elimination of excess fluids. It is particularly useful for hastening the healing of wounds.

In addition, gotu kola is considered "food for the brain." As such, it is said to combat stress and depression, energize flagging mental powers, fight senility, ward off a nervous breakdown, and improve reflexes.

DESCRIPTION AND PARTS USED

Gotu kola is a perennial plant native to India, Ceylon (Sri Lanka), China, Indonesia, Australia, the South Pacific, Madagascar, and some parts of Africa. It prefers tropical temperatures and damp, swampy areas, but can flourish in rocky, sunny areas up to 2,000 feet.

Gotu kola's appearance changes, depending on growing conditions. In shallow water, the plant puts forth floating roots and the leaves rest on top of the water. In dry locations, it puts out numerous small roots and the leaves are small and thin. The entire plant is used medicinally.

HISTORICAL NOTES

Gotu kola has been used as medicine in the Ayurvedic tradition of India for thousands of years. It is listed in the historic *Susruta Samhita*, an ancient Hindu medical text. It was also used extensively by the people of Java and other Indonesian islands.

In China, gotu kola is one of the reported "miracle elixirs of life," a reputation stemming from a healer of ancient times named LiChing Yun, who supposedly lived for 256 years. LiChing Yun's extraordinary longevity was attributed to his lifelong use of a tea brewed from gotu kola and other herbs. Gotu kola is prominently mentioned in the *Shennong Herbal*, which was compiled in China over 2,000 years ago.

SCIENTIFIC FINDINGS

Studies show gotu kola has a positive effect on the circulatory system. It seems to improve the flow of blood while strengthening the veins and tiny capillaries. It has been used successfully to treat phlebitis, leg cramps, and abnormal tingling of the extremities. Gotu kola is considered particularly helpful for those who are bedridden or confined to a wheelchair.

Gotu kola has demonstrated impressive clinical results in reducing some types of scarring, especially when applied during the inflammatory period of the wound. In patients with second- and third-degree burns, an extract of gotu kola gave excellent results if treatment was begun immediately after the accident. Daily local applications to the affected area and intramuscular injections limited shrinking of the skin as it healed, prevented infection, and inhibited scar formation.

TRADITIONAL USE

Internal. In the Ayurvedic tradition, the advice is to take 1/2 cup of tea 3 times daily for at least 1 month. Brew the tea using 1 level teaspoonful (1/6 ounce or 4 grams) of the herb per 8 ounces of freshly boiled water.

External. To treat nervous disorders the Ayurvedic way, Brahmi (gotu kola) oil is applied externally all over the entire body, including the scalp. If you wish to prepare this ancient remedy in the traditional way, you must make it with sesame oil. To prepare the oil, place a quantity of gotu kola parts in a jar and add cold-pressed sesame oil until the herb is awash. Cover and allow the oil to stand in a warm place for 14 days. Strain through cheesecloth to remove the exhausted herb parts, and the oil is ready to use. (For more information on preparing herbal oils, see Chapter 3.)

CONSIDERATIONS

Gotu kola is considered to be generally well tolerated when taken internally. The topical application of gotu kola salve has been reported to cause contact dermatitis, although very infrequently.

Green Tea *(Camellia sinensis)*

Worldwide, more people take tea than any other beverage, except water. Green tea is one of the sipping teas, so ancient its use as a refreshing drink dates back 5,000 years. If your primary interest is in the simple drinking of green tea for the pleasure it offers, please refer to Chapter 1, Traditional Sipping Teas. It's true that green tea is traditionally taken as a beverage, not as a medicinal tea, but times are changing.

Today, green tea is heralded as highly beneficial. The latest research shows that drinking green tea not only wards off heart disease, lowers the incidence of stroke, reduces the risk of cancer, brings down high blood pressure, and combats cold and flu symptoms, it even fights dental decay and bad breath.

DESCRIPTION AND PARTS USED

All sipping teas—green tea, oolong, and black tea (which includes the pekoes)—come from the same plant, *Camellia sinensis*. The parts used are the leaves. (For more information, see page 10.)

HISTORICAL NOTES

The history of *Camellia sinensis* is fully explored in Chapter 1. Because Part II is devoted to the healing qualities of various teas, let's proceed directly to the astounding new findings that support the use of green tea for its medicinal properties.

SCIENTIFIC FINDINGS

Green tea is rich in plant chemicals called polyphenols that are lost in the fermenting process other teas undergo. Polyphenols are antioxidants, the very substances science has determined help defuse free radicals, the compounds that roam the body causing all kinds of havoc. Free radicals are highly unstable and transfer their energy to the fats in cell membranes, disrupting the membranes and leading to disease. Free radicals are tied to premature aging and a whole list of diseases. The most important of the polyphenols in green tea is epigallocatechin gallate, or EGCG. Research indicates that EGCG is a powerful antioxidant—considered a stronger antioxidant than either vitamin E or C—with medicinal properties. As such, it provides very real preventive benefits. Here's a brief look at some of the clues that led to this conclusion:

• More people sip green tea in Japan than in any other country in the entire world. Dietary studies in Japan show that simply drinking four to six cups of green tea every day provides amazing protection against a host of killer diseases, as well as some nagging health problems that plague the whole world.

• Recent findings confirm that those Japanese who regularly drink green tea have a much lower incidence of various types of malignant tumors, including those found in the liver, pancreas, breast, esophagus, skin, and even, astoundingly, lungs. That's in spite of the fact that the majority of Japanese are addicted to smoking. In 1991, researchers connected with the American Cancer Society reported that Japanese cigarette smokers who regularly took green tea had a 45 percent lower risk of developing lung cancer than their countrymen who did not drink green tea.

• A double blind study in Europe indicated that drinking two cups of green tea each day can help decrease excess body fat. The tea will not, however, cause weight loss in someone who does not have *excess* fat.

• Green tea also fosters a healthy heart. One of the factors that contributes to coronary heart disease is plaque that attaches to artery walls and inhibits the flow of blood. An additional risk factor is the possibility of blood clots developing that can break free, lodge in an artery, and stop the flow of blood entirely. Green tea helps inhibit the production of platelets that cause the blood to thicken and clump into clots.

• Another factor implicated in heart disease is high blood pressure. Some prescription drugs that help lower blood pressure work by inhibiting an enzyme known as ACE (angiotension-converting enzyme). ACE, produced by the kidneys, causes blood vessels to constrict. Scientists have determined that green tea also inhibits the secretion of ACE. In a recent three-month study of thirty-seven people with high blood pressure, it was found that drinking green tea reduced blood pressure, on average, from 135 over 85 to 124 over 77.

• Yet another study compared the risk of stroke in green tea drinkers with those who chose other beverages. The subjects involved in this study were 6,000 nondrinking and nonsmoking Japanese women. It was determined that those who regularly took five cups of green tea daily cut by half their risk of suffering a stroke.

• In Japan, green tea, or an extract of the active constituents, is prescribed by doctors to treat viral influenza, as well as the common cold. Japanese studies show that even at concentrations as low as one part per million, an extract of EGCG controls the flu virus. And the good news is that the polyphenols in just one cup of green tea are 1,000 times more powerful than the extract.

• As far as dental health goes, green tea comes up a winner yet again. It has been shown to fight the bacteria that cause cavities and tartar. Finally, the *Journal of the Japanese Society of Food Science and Technology* has reported that green tea also slows the growth of the bacteria that contribute to bad breath or halitosis.

• Quick! Put the kettle on. Even if green tea isn't one of your favorites, the scientific data on green tea as both healer and preventive is just too strong to ignore. Green tea is very bitter, but don't let that put you off. It's quite easy to acquire a taste for this tea. Resting the water until it stops rolling helps reduce bitterness. So does a short steeping time.

TRADITIONAL USE

Internal. To brew green tea, use 1 teaspoon of loose tea or one tea bag per cup of tea. Heat water to boiling. Then take the water off the heat and let it stand a moment until it stops bubbling before pouring it over the tea. Cover and steep from 2 to 5 minutes. (For more information on brewing teas, see Chapter 3.)

CONSIDERATIONS

People have been drinking green tea for pleasure for centuries with no ill effects. Today, we know that green tea qualifies as one of the best healing teas in the history of the world. Enjoy.

Horehound *(Marrubium vulgare)*

Horehound is the herb you want to have on hand when you have asthma, a cough, a sore throat, or a cold. This noteworthy expectorant helps liquify mucus in the bronchial tubes and lungs, eases a cough, and soothes and coats a sore throat. It also helps relieve the dragged-out feeling that so often accompanies a bad cold. It even fights intestinal gas, helps against jaundice, and is a traditional remedy for intestinal worms.

DESCRIPTION AND PARTS USED

Horehound is a perennial that flourishes in the wild, prefers a warm, sunny location, isn't fussy about climate, and doesn't mind poor soil of low fertility. This herb is bushy and produces branching stems from one to two feet in height. It has white flowers and wrinkled "hairy" leaves that give the plant a wooly appearance. The leaves and tiny top flowers contain the medicinal properties.

HISTORICAL NOTES

This ancient herb has been used for centuries to flavor candy, cure colds, fight jaundice, and counteract toxins. Horehound was used by the Egyptians, Romans, and Greeks. Greek physicians prescribed horehound for the bite of a mad dog, or hoar hound, hence its common name.

The most celebrated use for horehound is clearing the lungs. The English master herbalist Gerard wrote as follows: "Syrup made of the greene fresh leaves and sugar is a most singular remedie against coughing and wheezing of the lungs and doth wonderfully and above credit ease such as have been long sicke of any consumption of the lungs, as hath beene often proved by the learned physitions of our London College."

Another master herbalist of the times, Culpeper, wrote, "It helpeth to expectorate tough phlegm from the chest, being taken with the roots of the Irris or Orris. There is a syrup made of this plant which I would recommend as an excellent help to evacuate tough phlegm and cold rheum from the lungs of aged persons, especially those who are asthmatic and short winded." Culpeper went further with his remarks: "Horehound purges away yellow jaundice; and, with the oil of roses, being dropped into the ears, eases the pain of them."

In some parts of England, this herb is still brewed into Horehound Ale, a healthful and appetizing beverage. The Latin name of this herb is believed to derive from the Hebrew *marrob*, meaning "bitter juice." The experts say horehound is one of the ancient bitter herbs the Jews use during the Feast of Passover.

SCIENTIFIC FINDINGS

Horehound offers vitamins A, B complex, C, E, and F, as well as volatile oils, resins, tannins, iron, and potassium. It also contains marrubiin, a bitter substance with healing properties.

Horehound
Cough & Cold Syrup

If you wish to make a very effective cough syrup and cold remedy that was a staple in medicine closets long ago, here's how to do it:

1/4 cup dried horehound parts
1 cup water
2 cups honey

1. *Boil horehound parts in the water for 10 minutes. Remove from heat and let the mixture rest for 5 minutes. Strain out the exhausted herb parts by pouring the liquid through cheesecloth.*

2. *Add honey and stir until it is smoothly combined with the herb mixture. Pour into a glass jar. Store at room temperature.*

Directions for Use

Dispense the horehound syrup by the tablespoonful as needed to ease a cough and comfort a cold sufferer.

TRADITIONAL USE

Internal. A cup of healing horehound tea, which actually tastes quite pleasant, is a good way to counteract the nasty effects of a cold. Pour 8 ounces of freshly boiled water over 7 1/4 teaspoons (1 ounce or 28.35 grams) of the dried herb. Cover, steep five minutes, strain, and sip hot. (For more information on brewing teas, see Chapter 3.) Sweeten with honey, if you like. Take 3 cups daily.

External. According to Culpeper, Horehound: "outwardly cleanses and abates the swollen part and pains that come by pricking thornes. With vinegar, it cleanses and heals tetters." In case you don't know what a "tetter" is, it's a rash that occurs on the palms of the hands, making them sore to the touch. If you have a tetter, see Chapter 3 for preparing a wash to ease it.

CONSIDERATIONS

Horehound is remarkably free of any adverse effects.

Horsetail *(Equisetum arvense)*

A diuretic and stiptic, horehound is used in the treatment of bleeding wounds—inside and out—kidney stones, urinary tract infections, cystitis, intestinal disorders, rheumatism, and gout. It increases circulation and helps the body use calcium more efficiently, thereby helping heal broken bones and strengthening connective tissues. Horsetail has been used for centuries as an aid to healthy hair, nails, bones, teeth, and skin.

DESCRIPTION AND PARTS USED

Horsetail has no leaves, no branches, and looks more like a little pine tree than anything else. It seldom attains a height greater than three feet and even finds a home in hard clay. These clumps of wild horsetail are said to be particularly valuable medicinally as the plant draws nutrients from the clay itself. Horsetail likes wet feet and is often found growing wild in fields and wet meadows. An old wive's tail says the presence of horsetail is a dead giveaway pointing to underground water. Wells have been dug on the strength of that belief.

HISTORICAL NOTES

Horsetail's botanical name relates to its appearance and is easy to explain. *Equisetum* comes from the Latin word *equus* meaning horse, and *seta* meaning bristle.

Several species of horsetail have been used medicinally since early Roman times. One old manuscript says, "It will heal sinews, though they be cut in sunder." Culpeper assures us, "It be very powerful to stop bleeding, either inward or outward. It also heals inward ulcers and solders together the tops of green wounds and cures all ruptures in children. The juice is of service in inflamings and all breakings-out of the skin. The decoction taken in wine helps stones and the tea strengthens the intestines and is effectual in a cough."

Horsetail, sometimes called the "scouring brush," contains silica, an abrasive. In ages past, horsetail stems were used by scullery maids in great houses to clean and polish the pewter dishes of the gentry. Dairymaids scoured their milk pails with horsetail. Fine cabinetmakers often smoothed and polished their work with the stems as well.

SCIENTIFIC FINDINGS

Horsetail contains calcium, copper, fatty acids, fluorine, selenium, nicotine, aconitic acid, equisitine, PABA, sodium, starch, vitamin B, and zinc. Numerous studies have confirmed that horsetail tea helps fractured bones heal faster and knit more smoothly. However, this is one powerful herb; it has been determined that excessive use can irritate the kidneys and intestines.

TRADITIONAL USE

Internal. Two weeks of treatment with horsetail tea should be followed by a week of rest. The treatment can be repeated, if necessary. Brew horsetail tea by pouring 8 ounces of freshly boiled water over 3 3/4 teaspoons (1/2 ounce or 14.175 grams) of the dried herb. Cover and steep for 3 minutes. (For more information on brewing teas, see Chapter 3.)

External. To inhibit external bleeding and help heal wounds, prepare and apply a horsetail poultice according to the instructions given in Chapter 3. One herbal I consulted says that bathing in water enriched with horsetail is an effective treatment for sluggish circulation, chilblains, rheumatism, and gout. If you wish to try what sounds like a pleasant experience, please see Chapter 3 for instructions on preparing an herbal bath.

CONSIDERATIONS

To avoid irritating your kidneys and intestines, do not use horsetail tea for any longer than two weeks in a row.

Ipe Roxo *(Tabebuia avellanedae)*

See Pau d'Arco.

Kombucha *(Fungus Japonicus)*

At this writing, kombucha tea, brewed from an unusual mushroom-type fungus, is enjoying an unprecedented surge of popularity in the United States. Kombucha tea is widely used today in Germany, France, Russia, Hawaii, and Asia. Not surprisingly, its origins have been traced back to China, the birthplace of all teas. In its most recent reincarnation, kombucha tea has been popping up all over the place. Articles have appeared in such publications as *USA Today* and *People*. The brew has been featured in major newspapers, and respected television news shows have done segments on it as well.

According to many reports—primarily anecdotal—kombucha tea boosts the immune system, increases energy levels, fights cancer and AIDS, eases arthritis and rheumatism, rids the body of toxins, normalizes blood pressure, reduces cholesterol levels, inhibits the aging process, lengthens the lifespan, eliminates acne, erases wrinkles, turns gray hair back to its original color, and stimulates hair growth.

DESCRIPTION AND PARTS USED

Although the kombucha is termed a "mushroom," it doesn't look very much like any mushroom you're likely to find in a produce market. Visualize a pancake about a half-inch-thick, ranging from six to ten inches wide. Color it a rich shade of coffee well-diluted with cream, then give it a glossy and glistening, slick and smooth top, and you'll come close.

But put away your knife and fork. This mushroom isn't for eating. When properly cared for, this friendly living organism not only produces a drinkable brew, it also produces a baby every week that can be used to start a new batch of tea.

Kombucha Tea

A few health-food stores offer the prepared beverage. However, if you wish to brew kombucha tea at home, consider the following recipe, derived from instructions that appeared in "The Outlook" on February 23, 1995. Betsy Pryor and Norman Bakers, partners in the enterprise, ship starter-mushrooms to clients all across the United States. If you wish to purchase one, the cost (including overnight shipping) is $50.00. (You'll find Laurel Farms' address and phone number in the Sources of Information section in the back of this book.) Legend has it that the kombucha should be given away freely and must not be sold. However, unless you know someone who's willing to part with a baby, buying a starter-mushroom may be the only way to get one.

This recipe will yield about 1 quart of kombucha tea. If you take 12 ounces of tea every day, which is the recommended amount, you'll need to prepare 2 batches of tea per week.

3 quarts distilled water
1 cup white sugar
4 tea bags, green or black
4 ounces apple cider vinegar

1. *Boil the distilled water in a large stainless steel pot. Add the sugar and boil for 5 minutes.*

2. *Add the tea bags. Remove from heat, cover, and let steep for 10 minutes. Remove the tea bags.*

3. *Cool the tea to room temperature, then pour into a 3- or 4-quart clear glass bowl. Don't use crystal, metal, ceramic, or plastic, and don't use a jar, not even a large one. The mushroom needs a large "breathing" space.*

4. *If you are brewing your first batch of tea, add 4 ounces of apple cider vinegar to the cooled liquid. If you have brewed tea before, omit the vinegar and add 4 ounces of previously prepared tea as a "starter" instead.*

5. Before handling the kombucha mushroom, it's best to remove your rings. No metal should touch the mushroom. Place it with the rough, darker side down, smooth side up, on top of the tea. Cover the bowl with cheesecloth or a clean white T-shirt cut to size. Cross two strips of tape over the cloth and onto the glass, and secure with a rubber band.

6. Place in a dark, quiet, ventilated place in which the temperature is 70–90°F. Let rest for 7 to 10 days. Remove the mother mushroom with a wooden or plastic spoon (do not use metal). There will be a "baby" mushroom on top. Separate the baby from the mother by pulling apart gently.

7. Using the cover cloth as a strainer, pour the newly fermented tea from the bowl into a glass or plastic container. Refrigerate the tea.

Recipe courtesy of Laurel Farms of Studio City, California.

HISTORICAL NOTES

The first recorded use of kombucha tea occurred in China during the Tsin Dynasty in 221 B.C. Back then, it was known as "The Remedy for Immortality" or "The Divine Tsche." During the following centuries, what some call the "magic mushroom" traveled from China to Korea. There are two versions of how the tea came to be called "Kombucha." First, various articles say that in 414 B.C., a healer by the name of Dr. Kombu—nationality unknown—carried the fungus to Japan where the mushroom tea became known as *Kombu-cha* in his honor. *Cha*, of course, means tea. Second, and perhaps more credible, other sources identify *kombu* as a type of Japanese seaweed, hence *kombu-cha*.

Although it is variously called "Manchurian tea," "Fungus japonicus" (in Japan), "Champignon de longue vie" or "mushroom of long life" (in France), and Kargasok tea (for a region of Russia where the brew is much favored), it is best known as "kombucha tea" today.

SCIENTIFIC FINDINGS

Little research has been done in the United States. Most of the data isn't even available in English, having been reported in various German publications. The work of Dr. Rudolph Sklenar, a physician who died in 1987, is often cited today by those who wish to extol the benefits of the tea. Dr. Sklenar began using kombucha tea in the 1960s to treat cancer patients. Unfortunately, his reports are discounted by the medical and scientific communities. According to the popular press, however, components that have been identified in the fermented brew include glucuronic acid (reported to be a good liver detoxifier), hyaluronic acid (found in connective tissue), chondroitin sulfate (found in cartilage), yeast enzymes, lactic acid, usnic acid (an organic acid that occurs in lichens), and an array of B vitamins. And there are many today who swear to the healthful and energizing effects of this tea.

TRADITIONAL USE

Internal. Drink 4 ounces of kombucha tea (see recipe on page 159) 3 times a day, before or after meals. Some have likened the taste of this tea to Moselle, a dry white wine, but it tastes more like apple cider to me. Most people seem to agree.

CONSIDERATIONS

Although no explanation is given, all articles on kombucha tea state that it should not be taken by pregnant women or nursing mothers.

LaPacho *(Tabebuia avellanedae)*

See Pau d'Arco.

Licorice *(Glycyrrhiza glabra)*

Licorice is highly beneficial to the entire gastrointestinal tract. It fights nausea, helps sweeten a sour stomach, cleanses the colon, supports the liver, and is the herbalist's treatment of choice for colitis, diverticulosis, and gastritis. Licorice is a noted expectorant and anti-inflammatory that helps liquify mucus, making it valuable against colds, sore throats, bronchitis, sinus and lung congestion. It is considered helpful in cases of PMS, allergies, hypoglycemia, stress, and muscular and skeletal spasms. Licorice has even proven effective against herpes simplex when used topically.

DESCRIPTION AND PARTS USED

Licorice is a perennial shrub that grows from three to seven feet high. It prefers a temperate climate and puts forth long, cylindrical, branched, flexible roots that send forth runners every which way. The valuable properties of licorice are found in both the runners and roots, which are harvested in the fall. Licorice root is not used fresh; it is dried to lock in its medicinal properties.

HISTORICAL NOTES

Licorice is one of the most ancient medicinals in the Chinese pharmacopoeia. The medical use of licorice in Eastern culture dates back at least 4,000 years. The 2,000-year-old *Shennong Herbal*, which includes more than 365 plant drugs, lists licorice as a "superior" drug.

SCIENTIFIC FINDINGS

Licorice is one of the most extensively investigated of all botanical medicines. Because of its pharmacological activity, it is useful in a wide range of health conditions. It has been established that licorice is: anti-inflammatory; antiallergic; antibacterial; antiviral, antifungal; antimicrobial; antihepatotoxic; anticonvulsive; and immunostimulatory. In short, licorice helps minimize injury, while boosting the immune system at the same time. Licorice also exerts a unique normalizing action on estrogen metabolism, inhibiting estrogen action when levels are too high and stimulating estrogen action when levels are too low.

Licorice has a long history of successful use in the treatment of peptic, gastric, and duodenal ulcers. In the treatment of ulcers, licorice does not slow down the production of gastric acid. Instead, it steps up the defenses that prevent an ulcer from forming in the first place. This action includes increasing the number of protective mucus-secreting cells, improving the quality of the mucus produced, increasing the life span of the intestinal cells, and enhancing the strength of the gastrointestinal tract lining. However, researchers have unearthed a harmful side effect that occurs with overuse of this herb.

There are several components of licorice. One, carbenoxolone, has antiulcer action. Another, glycyrrhetic acid, has the potential to cause high blood pressure. This acid fosters the buildup of sodium and simultaneously reduces the amount of potassium circulating in the bloodstream. It also causes the body to retain water. Scientists solved the problem by creating deglycyrrhizinated licorice or DGL. If you are considering the use of licorice for the treatment of ulcers, please talk to your doctor about DGL. It has racked up some impressive results in double-blind studies.

TRADITIONAL USE

Internal. If you are using the powdered form of whole licorice root to brew a healing tea, limit yourself to 3 cups of tea daily, using 1/4 teaspoon (.035 ounces or 1 gram) of powder per 8 ounces of freshly boiled water. (For more information on brewing teas, see Chapter 3.) If you are using the root itself, please see Chapter 3 for instructions on brewing a decoction.

External. Clinical studies have shown that glycyrrhizin, when used as a soothing wash, can be helpful in reducing the healing time and pain associated with oral and genital herpes lesions. Glycyrrhizin inactivates the herpes simplex virus and stimulates the synthesis and release of interferon, one of the defensive elements of the immune system. If you are using licorice root (and not the powdered form), a decoction is called for. To treat herpes simplex, please see Chapter 3 for information on brewing a strong decoction.

CONSIDERATIONS

Although studies show not everyone reacts the same way, the ingestion of large doses of licorice can cause high sodium and low potassium levels in blood. Licorice should not be used by anyone with high blood pressure, with the potential to develop high blood pressure, or with kidney problems. Do not use licorice if you are taking heart medication.

You should know that studies have shown individuals who normally consume a healthy diet of foods rich in potassium (fruits and vegetables) and restrict their salt intake, which we all should be doing anyway, remain free of the side effects associated with the acidic component of glycyrrhizin.

Lobelia *(Lobelia inflata)*

Lobelia is traditionally used in the treatment of colds, sore throats, laryngitis, asthma, bronchitis, and even pneumonia. It takes down a fever and is a noted relaxant and cough suppressant. Lobelia also helps people break the smoking habit.

DESCRIPTION AND PARTS USED

Lobelia, also known as Indian tobacco, is an annual plant indigenous to the eastern half of the United States. This plant has an erect, hairy stem and grows up to three feet tall. Each stem has numerous oval-shaped leaves. From July through October, lobelia puts forth bluish flowers, which give way to seed-bearing fruits. The parts used medicinally are those appearing above ground.

HISTORICAL NOTES

From all accounts, lobelia was known medicinally to Native Americans and was used extensively by the early colonists. In 1813, Samuel Thomson, a self-taught doctor of New Hampshire, discovered that his prescriptions for herbal medicines, including lobelia, were so valuable they were being appropriated by other doctors. Accordingly, Thomson had his formulas patented, thus starting the era of patent medicines. In 1822, Thomson produced an 800-page manual of plant drugs that he marketed at the price of $20.00, a huge sum in those days. Of Lobelia, he wrote: "There is no vegetable which the earth produces more harmless in its effect on the human system, and none more powerful in removing disease and promoting health than Lobelia." Of the 65 major plants listed in Thomson's manual, at least 50 species are still considered valuable today.

Thomson's life was full of lawsuits, including one involving lobelia. A patient died after Thomson administered this herb. He was subsequently sued by the family but was found not guilty. Soon after that, lobelia appeared in the *United States Pharmacopoeia* as a reputable drug.

SCIENTIFIC FINDINGS

Many studies have shown that lobelia is a very effective expectorant. It helps liquify the secretions of the respiratory tract, making it easier to cough them up and out, thus restoring free breathing. Lobelia stimulates the adrenal gland to release the hormones that cause the bronchial muscles to relax. This herb is considered an effective aid for those who are addicted to any form of tobacco. Lobeline, a constituent of lobelia, has many of the same pharmacological actions as nicotine but is regarded as less powerful. Because lobeline mimics nicotine, lobelia tea can be an effective means of reducing the discomfort of nicotine withdrawal by those who wish to give up smoking (or chewing) tobacco.

TRADITIONAL USE

Internal. To brew lobelia tea, use no more than 1/2 gram of the dried herb spread out over 3 doses daily. (For more information on brewing teas, see Chapter 3)

External. Lobelia is an excellent relaxant and antispasmodic. To relieve muscle spasms, lobelia can be used as a poultice, a fomentation, or an additive to bath water. To prepare any of these, please see Chapter 3.

Winter Tonic

It is written that this formula is useful for the treatment of coldness, negative emotional states, weakness, irregular menstruation, and menstrual cramps. It is also considered useful for those, be they male or female, who suffer from muscle cramps.

Two of the herbal ingredients—cramp bark (Viburnum opulus) and squawvine (Mitchella repens) are not mentioned elsewhere in this book. They are noteworthy because of their antispasmodic properties. A well-stocked herb shop should be able to supply both these herbs.

It seems pretty obvious that the real warming action of this old-time Winter Tonic comes as much from the wine used in the brewing as it does from the herbal content. In a drafty house heated only by a log or coal fire in a fireplace, I expect each tiny sip was very welcome.

2 parts raspberry leaves
2 parts cramp bark
2 parts angelica root
2 parts squawvine
1 part chamomile
1 part ginger root
1 part lobelia
1 quart good quality red wine (Port is traditional, but you may substitute any rich red wine of your choice.)

1. *Assemble and blend all the herbs.*

2. *Put the wine into an enameled saucepan. Measure out 6 ounces of the combined herbs and stir them into the wine. Cover the pot and heat gently just until the wine begins to simmer. Do not permit the mixture to boil. (If you wish to eliminate the alcohol content of the tonic, uncover the pot and let the mixture bubble for 5 minutes or so. This method will allow you to retain the medicinal qualities of the herbs and all the flavor of the wine, but the alcohol will evaporate as the brew boils.)*

3. *Cover and let the blend stand for 24 hours. Strain off the exhausted herb parts and bottle the tonic.*

Directions for Use:
Take 1 tablespoonful of this warming Winter Tonic 3 times daily, 20 minutes before meals.

CONSIDERATIONS

The ingestion of too much lobelia usually causes violent vomiting, an example of the protection built into herbs by Mother Nature. If toxic levels were ingested and retained, symptoms of nicotine poisoning would ensue, starting with dizziness and nausea and progressing all the way to respiratory failure.

Do not exceed recommended dosage as discussed in Traditional Use. I don't expect you'll ever need to know this, but the antidote for acute poisoning is 2 mg of atropine given subcutaneously.

Mahuang *(Ephedra sinica)*

Mahuang is an effective decongestant and bronchodilator with marked anti-inflammatory properties. It's also a good expectorant. As such, it is traditionally used as a treatment for asthma, bronchitis, allergies, sinusitis, and the common cold. Mahuang is also a mild diuretic and fever reducer that has proven very valuable against hypotension (low blood pressure). Of particular interest to many is this herb's ability to suppress the appetite, stimulate metabolism, and bring about substantial weight loss.

According to Chinese physicians—and they've been prescribing mahuang for thousands of years—the herb must only be used by those with a strong yang constitution. It is considered too stimulating and too powerful for anyone who is weak, exhausted, and low in energy.

DESCRIPTION AND PARTS USED

All the *Ephedra* species are upright shrubs that typically grow from one and a half to four feet tall. They have many erect yellow-green branches coming from a slender central trunk. Found throughout the world, *Ephedra* prefers an arid desert climate. Mahuang, the most powerful of the species, is indigenous to Asia, but varieties of *Ephedra* are found in Europe, North America, India, and Pakistan. The parts used are the stems and branches.

HISTORICAL NOTES

The medicinal use of mahuang in China dates from approximately 2800 B.C. to the present, but it wasn't until 1923 that practitioners of Western medicine became interested in this herb. That's when scientists identified, isolated, and began experimenting with mahuang's principal alkaloid, ephedrine. It took another four years before ephedrine was successfully synthesized. Since then, both ephedrine and pseudoephedrine, also found in mahuang, have been used extensively in prescription drugs and over-the-counter cold-relievers, decongestants, and allergy medications.

SCIENTIFIC FINDINGS

Ephedrine's action is very like that of epinephrine (adrenaline). It's much less active, but it works for a longer period of time and has a more pronounced effect on the brain and nervous system. In short, ephedrine relaxes the bronchial muscles, the muscles of the airways, and even the muscles of the uterus. It also increases blood flow through the heart, brain and muscles, but at the expense of kidney and intestinal blood flow. As a bronchodilator, the herb's peak effect occurs in one hour and lasts about five hours.

Studies with both humans and animals show that ephedrine really will help in weight loss. It has an appetite-suppressant effect, but mainly it works by increasing the metabolic rate and assisting in fat breakdown. Research shows that weight reduction is greatest in individuals who have a naturally low basal metabolic rate.Used alone, mahuang was associated with losses of 14 percent in body weight and 42 percent in body fat. The best results were achieved when mahuang was taken in combination with caffeine or theophylline, a white crystalline powder that dilates blood vessels. In those subjects, there was a loss of 25 percent in body weight and 75 percent in body fat. Green tea (*Camellia sinensis*), reviewed earlier, contains the necessary theophylline (plus some caffeine), and is a healing tea in its own right.

TRADITIONAL USE

Internal. If you are preparing tea using the dried herb, a dose of

500 to 1,000 mg taken 2 or 3 times a day is the recommended amount for asthma and weight loss. (For more information on brewing tea, see Chapter 3.) If your aim is to drop some pounds, don't forget to take green tea, too.

CONSIDERATIONS

Ephedrine, the principal component of mahuang, can increase blood pressure and heart rate, and cause insomnia and anxiety. It should not be taken by individuals with heart disease, high blood pressure, thyroid disease, diabetes, or an enlarged prostate. It must not be taken by patients on antihypertensives or antidepressants.

Mahuang is a very powerful herb, for occasional use only. Don't be afraid of it, but don't abuse it either.

Marigold

See Calendula.

Marshmallow *(Althea officinalis)*

Marshmallow is a soothing, healing demulcent, considered valuable for all lung ailments, including asthma. It has been used for centuries to soothe sore throats, ease a cough, and treat ulcers and diseases of the gastrointestinal tract. It is particularly useful against irritations caused by diarrhea and dysentery. Marshmallow is also an excellent anti-inflammatory that helps relieve swollen and irritated joints.

DESCRIPTION AND PARTS USED

Many varieties of the mallow species grow well in home gardens and are a valuable addition to any herbal plot. The small-leafed mallow has long, slender stems, rounded toothed leaves, and small pale pink or lavender flowers. Its round fruits are known as "cheeses." Country-bred children sometimes eat them when serving them to their dolls as a tea-party delicacy.

The leaves and roots are harvested in autumn and the brown outer covering is removed. The whitish inner core is the source of the demulcent substance and was once used to make marshmallows. Today, a bag of marshmallows contains nothing but sugar, gelatin, and preservatives.

HISTORICAL NOTES

During his reign, King Charlemagne (A.D. 742–814) decreed that the marsh mallow be planted throughout his kingdom to ensure an abundant supply. Perhaps the king had ulcers and wanted this soothing herb on hand.

About 800 years after Charlemagne's death, master herbalist Culpeper described the "bloody flux" from which his son suffered. The London College of Physicians called this dread disease "the plague in the guts." Many died from it. However, Culpeper wrote in his journal that his son was healed after just two days on the "Mallow cure." As treatment, Culpeper gave the boy, "Mallow bruised and boyled in milke and drinke."

The experts say marshmallow seeds, being a plant of the salt marshes, probably arrived in America as part of the dried straw packing used to cushion fragile imports.

SCIENTIFIC FINDINGS

All the mallows have mucilaginous properties. In pharmacological lingo, this refers to substances that absorb water, swell, and form a viscous fluid. Mucilage forms a fine layer on the surface of a mucous membrane, thereby protecting it from irritants, soothing any inflammation, and giving the body an opportunity to heal the affected area. Mucilage is not absorbed into the body, so its effects are always purely local. In other words, marshmallow tea will soothe a sore throat and relieve a cough caused by irritation in the throat, but it won't do a thing to cure a cough or sore throat arising from a systemic infection.

TRADITIONAL USE

Internal. Heat destroys the mucilaginous properties of this herb. To brew a healing mallow tea, make a cold infusion by soaking 1 heaping tablespoonful (1/2 ounce or 14.175 grams) of the herb overnight in 6 ounces of cold water. Warm the infusion slightly the following day and strain off the exhausted herb parts. Drink 2 to 3 cups throughout the day. (For more information on preparing a cold infusion, see Chapter 3.)

External. Mallow root, powdered or well-crushed, "may be relied upon to remove the most obstinate inflammation and prevent mortification," or so says an old herbal. For instructions on preparing a poultice, please see Chapter 3. If you want to try one of the old ways of preparing a mallow poultice, simply save the herbal residue left over from the cold infusion, warm slightly, slather the damp herbs on a piece of white bread and apply herb-side down to the affected part.

CONSIDERATIONS

The mallows are mild in action and free of unwanted side effects.

Milk Thistle *(Silybum marianum)*

Milk thistle is the time-honored treatment for all liver disorders, including cirrhosis, jaundice, and hepatitis. This herb contains silymarin, a potent flavonoid that fights free radical damage and exerts a protective effect on the liver (and kidneys). Milk thistle even stimulates the production of new liver cells.

DESCRIPTION AND PARTS USED

The milk thistle can be an annual or biennial, depending on climate. It grows naturally in dry, rocky soils in southern and western Europe and some parts of the United States. The branched stem attains a height of one to three feet and bears dark green, shiny leaves with spiny or scalloped edges that can be streaked with white along the veins. The plant puts forth one purple-red flower per stem; the plant is surrounded by sharp spines. The seeds, fruit, and leaves are all used for medicinal purposes.

HISTORICAL NOTES

Milk thistle was named for both its appearance, described above, and the original use to which it was put. In medieval times, milk thistle tea was given to nursing mothers to stimulate the production of milk and enrich the "formula." From all accounts, it was first used by early herbalists in Germany to induce lactation and then was found to be "wondrous beneficial" for liver complaints. As its fame spread, milk thistle became the "specific" for liver dysfunction.

SCIENTIFIC FINDINGS

Silybum marianum extracts, standardized to contain between 70 and 80 percent silymarin, are widely used in European pharmaceutical drugs for liver complaints. The ability of this herb to prevent liver destruction and boost liver function has been determined to result from silymarin's inhibition of some toxins responsible for liver damage, plus its ability to stimulate the production of new liver cells to replace old or damaged cells.

Silymarin is a potent antioxidant that can neutralize free radicals, those tiny molecules that injure other molecules, and can contribute to liver and cell damage throughout the body. Silymarin is many times more potent as an antioxidant than the better-known vitamin E. Silymarin has been shown to increase the glutathione content of the liver by more than 35 percent. Glutathione is a chemical the body requires to detoxify a wide range of harmful substances. Simply increasing the glutathione output of the liver gives the body more ammunition against toxins.

In a double-blind clinical study, silymarin showed remarkable results on 129 patients with liver damage, various types of fatty degeneration of the liver, and chronic hepatitis. Another study of silymarin involving patients with liver damage due to alcohol, diabetes, viruses, or exposure to toxins racked up impressive results, including regenerative and restorative effects, confirmed by biopsy.

The protective effects of silymarin have been confirmed in other double-blind clinical studies. It was judged particularly effective in protecting against alcohol- and chemical-induced liver damage. Some evidence also indicates it is of value in cases of viral hepatitis.

Abnormal liver function is implicated in cases of psoriasis. Silymarin seems to be of value in the treatment of this skin condition because of its ability to improve liver function and inhibit the synthesis of leukotrienes, chemical compounds that cause allergic and inflammatory reactions.

TRADITIONAL USE

Internal. In the studies referred to above, 70 to 210 mg of silymarin was administered 3 times daily. There's no way to know the silymarin content of the dried herb, but 3 cups per day of a strongly-brewed healing tea should prove sufficient. Please see the box for recommended dosage or ask the advice of a knowledgeable staff member when purchasing loose herbs. For brewing instructions, please refer to Chapter 3.

CONSIDERATIONS

A large body of clinical evidence has been amassed in Europe where silymarin preparations are widely used. Results of the studies show a complete lack of toxicity. However, because milk thistle increases bile flow, expect a loose stool if taking this herb for a long period of time.

Mullein (*Verbascum thapsus*)

Mullein is a valuable decongestant that helps restore free breathing. It is a time-honored remedy for asthma, hay fever, and bronchitis and is a champion expectorant that loosens a dry, unproductive cough. In the process of clearing congestion, mullein soothes irritation in the throat and bronchial passages, too. As an antispasmodic, mullein can relieve stomach cramps and help control diarrhea; paradoxically, it is mildly laxative. This herb also acts to reduce glandular swellings and is a mild sedative that fights insomnia.

DESCRIPTION AND PARTS USED

Mullein is a striking looking plant that attains a height of four to eight feet by the time it's two years old. The first year, the plant develops large, wooly leaves that last through the winter. In the second year, this biennial puts forth a flower-studded spike of yellow blossoms that pushes up from a thick base of leftover leaves. The leaves develop along the entire length of the stalk, decreasing in size as they rise. This arrangment by Mother Nature causes the small top leaves to send raindrops down the entire length of the stem and all the way to the roots. Both the leaves and flowers have medicinal uses.

HISTORICAL NOTES

The tall stalks of mullein with yellow flowers at the tip not only look like lighted candles, but the ancients used them as torches. The medieval English master herbalist Parkinson tells us: "Verbascum is called of the Latines Candela regia, and Candelaria, because the elder age used the stalks dipped in suet to burne, whether at funeralls or otherwise."

Verbascum thapsus, known as the "great mullein," was imported from Europe because of its medicinal value. In ancient times, mullein was believed to be a sure safeguard against evil spirits and magic. Ulysses is said to have taken great mullein to protect against the wiles of Circe.

The ladies of ancient Rome used mullein tea to dye their hair golden blonde. A very old herbal says, "The golden floures of Mulleyn stiped in lye, causeth the heare to war yellow, being washed therewithall."

SCIENTIFIC FINDINGS

Mullein is called a "natural wonder" herb with sedative properties that are neither addictive nor poisonous. It has been determined that this plant has marked demulcent, emollient, and astringent properties. The substances found in this herb include choline, hesperidin, magnesium, PABA, saponins, sulfur, and vitamins B_2, B_5, B_{12}, and D.

TRADITIONAL USE

Internal. Mullein tea is easily made by steeping 1 tablespoon (1/2 ounce or 14.175 grams) of the dried herb in 8 ounces of freshly boiled hot water. (For more information on brewing teas, see Chapter 3.) Strain well. Take 1 to 2 cups of this healing tea daily. For lung congestion and stubborn coughs, many sources suggest smoking this herb. I suggest sipping the tea. Smoking anything is a bad idea.

External. Mullein oil is considered one of the best remedies for ear complaints that nature has to offer. Expert herbalists suggest applying a few drops in the affected ear and letting the herb work overnight. (Refer to Chapter 3 for directions on preparing an herbal-based oil.)

CONSIDERATIONS

None of the many sources I consulted lists any instances of reported toxicity. Mullein seems complete free of nasty surprises.

Parsley *(Petroselinum crispum)*

Parsley is a diuretic herb traditionally used to treat all cases of fluid retention, including edema and obesity. It helps get rid of the bloat that sometimes accompanies the menses and relieves certain menstrual disorders as well.

Parsley is wonderfully cleansing. It benefits the lungs, stomach, liver, and thyroid, and has repeatedly proved itself valuable against bladder infections. It helps in the removal of all stones, including gallstones, if they are not too large. In old Greece, parsley was called the "stone breaker."

DESCRIPTION AND PARTS USED

You probably know what parsley looks like—just about everyone is familiar with its curly leaves of intense green—but you may not know that this herb produces small yellow flowers. Parsley is indigenous to Turkey, Algeria, Sardinia, and Lebanon. All parts of the plant are useful, including the fruits, berries, stems, leaves, and roots.

HISTORICAL NOTES

The Romans became enamored of parsley during their travels and brought it to what is now England. Inhabitants of the area promptly adopted it and cultivated it. Colonists brought it to the New World.

The ancient Greeks used parsley medicinally, as well as to cleanse their breath of garlic and other odiferous foods. They also wove it into garlands to honor their best athletes. The Greeks wore these parsley crowns called "chaplets" during banquets in the belief that the fumes of the wine would be absorbed, thus preventing the wearer from becoming inebriated. Around 270 B.C., the Greek poet Theocretus wrote the following:

> At Sparta's palace, twenty beauteous maids
> The pride of Greece, fresh garlands crowned their heads
> With hyacinths and twining parsley drest
> Graced joyful Menelaus' marriage feast.

The medicinal uses credited to parsley throughout the ages are almost endless, but all agree on the diuretic and deobstruent properties of this herb. Master herbalist Parkinson wrote, "The rootes boiled into broth help open obstruction of the liver, veines, and other parts . . . The rootes likewise boyled with leg of mutton will have as their operation to cause urine." Fellow herbalist Gerard agreed. He wrote, "Parsley seed waste away winde, are good for suche as have dropsie, draw down the menses, bring away the afterbirth; they be commended also against the cough, if they be boyled or mixed for such a purpose . . . They be also goode to be put into clysters against the stone or torments of the gut."

Parsley seeds were once credited with magic powers. Eating

the seed was said to confer invisibility and supernatural strength on the consumer.

SCIENTIFIC FINDINGS

Parsley is so full of nutrients that it can be considered one of nature's preventive medicines. It is high in vitamin B and potassium, and rich in iron, chlorophyll, calcium, phosphorus, and vitamins A and C. This herb can, therefore, strengthen the body and help build resistance to infections and diseases. Parsley even contains a substance that scientists have determined inhibits the development of cancer cells. The jury is still out, but some believe parsley may yet prove to be a cancer preventive.

TRADITIONAL USE

Internal. Parsley tea taken after meals is good protection against indigestion. Simply steep a few sprigs of the curly green leaves and stems in freshly boiled water, and sip slowly. If you eat the wilted leaves, so much the better. Parsley tea can also be used to treat a urinary complaint.

When purchasing the dried herb for therapeutic use, find out what portion of the herb is included. The roots, for example, are much more powerful than the leaves. Follow the manufacturer's recommendations as to dosage.

External. One old herbal assures the reader that rubbing parsley oil on the scalp will stimulate hair growth. (See Chapter 3 for information on preparing herbal oils.)

CONSIDERATIONS

Pregnant women should not use parsley as it can bring on early labor. Nursing mothers should be aware that parsley can dry up the milk supply. However, remember that after a child is weaned parsley tea can be useful to inhibit milk production and relieve the discomfort of overfull breasts.

Parsley is a warming herb. Avoid using it when the body is battling acute infection or when inflammation is present, especially if the kidneys are involved.

Pau d'Arco *(Tabebuia avellanedae)*

Pau d'arco, pronounced pow-dar-co, is a heroic natural medicinal that reportedly fights cancer—including leukemia—tumors, AIDS, liver disease, rheumatism, diabetes, ulcers, allergies, and all types of infections. It has even proven useful against candidiasis (yeast infections), warts, and smoker's coughs.

DESCRIPTION AND PARTS USED

This handsome tree reaches for the sky. It can attain a height of 125 feet. Native to Brazil, pau d'arco has large trumpet-shaped rose to violet-colored flowers that bloom in profusion just before the new leaves appear in the spring. There are around 100 *Tabebuia* species native to tropical America, but this one—*T. avellanedae*—is the one with the power. The bark is the portion of the tree that is used medicinally.

HISTORICAL NOTES

Pau d'arco appears to be a corruption of a local name for one variety of *Tabebuia* called *Palo d'arco*, or "bow wood," by the natives. Brazilian Indians have used Pau d'arco bark for centuries against a host of ailments, including colitis, dysentery, diarrhea, constipation, bedwetting, fever, sore throat, snakebite, and cancers of the esophagus, intestines, lung, and prostate, as well as for respiratory problems, arthritis, poor circulation, and even syphilis.

SCIENTIFIC FINDINGS

Pau d'arco's medicinal uses and extracts of its active constituents have been studied for the past century. Interestingly enough, research shows that significantly better results are racked up by the whole bark than by the extracts. When the extracts are refined and individual chemicals taken from the whole herb are tested, effectiveness is seen to be diminished.

Pau d'arco's antibacterial, antiviral, antiparasitic, anticancer, and anti-inflammatory properties have been confirmed in scientific testing. One author summarizes its effects in these words:

> The spectrum of clinical applications of *T. avellanedae* is quite broad. Current use has focused on its anticancer and antimicrobial activity. Its use is extremely popular in the treatment of intestinal candidiasis and vaginal candidiasis (topically and internally). There are also many anecdotal reports of remission of different forms of cancer from the use of this botanical.

TRADITIONAL USE

Internal. The "fixings" for tea are variously called (and sold as) LaPacho, Taheebo, Tecoma, and Ipe Roxo. Because the medicinal qualities are found in the bark of this tree, it's necessary to prepare a decoction. Boil 1 teaspoon (1/6 ounce or 4 grams) of pau d'arco bark in 8 ounces of water for 5 to 15 minutes. Strain and sip. The standard dose is 1 cup of decocted bark 2 to 8 times per day. The above directions differ from the general instructions in Chapter 3 in that this bark must be well boiled to extract the herb's active properties. (For more information on preparing a decoction, see Chapter 3.)

External. To treat vaginitis, soak a tampon in a strong decoction. Insert the medicated tampon vaginally and change it every 24 hours until symptoms are eased.

CONSIDERATIONS

The scientific literature lists no reports of human toxicity when the whole bark is used as a decoction.

Peppermint *(Mentha piperita)*

Peppermint is a noted digestive aid that stimulates the salivary glands, helps eliminate nausea, eases heartburn, promotes burping, and calms stomach spasms and cramps. Because of its action on the gastric lining, peppermint actually shortens the amount of time food spends in the stomach. This herb is traditionally used to cleanse and strengthen the entire body, including the heart muscle. Because of its stimulating and warming properties, peppermint tea is a favorite old-time remedy for chills, colds, colic, and rheumatism. It can even help relieve the nauseated feeling that often accompanies a migraine or "sick" headache.

DESCRIPTION AND PARTS USED

Botanically speaking, peppermint is a hybrid that falls somewhere between spearmint and watermint. Most of the members of the mint family grow wild and like wet feet. Left on their own to choose their environment, these herbs favor the banks of brooks and streams or low damp meadows, but they do very well under cultivation as long as the soil is rich and moist. Of all the mints, peppermint is the most widely used. For the home-brewing of peppermint tea, the leaves and flowering tops are used.

HISTORICAL NOTES

Medical prescriptions inscribed on old papyrus scrolls give evidence that peppermint has been used in Egypt since ancient times. As an effective medicinal and flavorful culinary herb, mint is in common use in both Middle Eastern and Asian lands today.

The benefits of peppermint have been appreciated on this side of the ocean for a very long time, too. Peppermint has been listed in the *United States Pharmacopoeia* for more than 150 years.

SCIENTIFIC FINDINGS

Everyone is familiar with the taste of peppermint, so it shouldn't come as a surprise to learn that the herb contains menthol, along with volatile oils, menthone, methyl acetate, tannic acid, terpenes, and vitamin C. It has been determined that oil of peppermint has very strong antispasmodic action. This property alone makes it valuable for relieving pains in the digestive tract, as well as cramps in the abdomen. Pharmacists often use peppermint in compound medicines because of its well-known ability to make disagreeable-tasting drugs palatable.

TRADITIONAL USE

Internal. To brew a flavorful cup of peppermint tea, use 1 heaping teaspoon (1/6 ounce or 4 grams) of dried herb parts to 8 ounces of freshly boiled water. Steep, strain, and allow to cool. (For more information on brewing teas, see Chapter 3.) As a medicinal drink, peppermint tea is traditionally taken cold for the relief of nausea, headache, heartburn, and flatulence.

External. Several sources I consulted claim that the bruised fresh leaves have a slight anesthetic effect. To relieve localized pain, pluck a few fresh leaves from the peppermint thriving in your garden, crinkle them up, smooth them back out, and apply to the affected area.

CONSIDERATIONS

Peppermint is considered perfectly harmless. It may be used freely.

Propolis

Strictly speaking, propolis is not an herb, but it is a marvelous natural medicinal derived from the hives of honeybees. Propolis is traditionally used for coughs and colds. It fights the flu, can clear a sore throat overnight, and is valuable against prostate disease. With regular use, propolis is one of nature's premiere preventives. It strengthens the entire body and gives the immune system a boost, thereby helping to build resistance against infection and disease.

DESCRIPTION AND PARTS USED

Honeybees collect the shiny golden-brown resin from pine trees and carry it home, where it is treated to the "magic" of the bee and then mixed into wax. The result is propolis, one of those stunning products Mother Nature devised to protect her creatures. The bees plaster propolis all over the interior of the hive and use it to line brood cells, it disinfects and protects against contamination, insuring that the hive remains disease-free. When harvested by the beekeeper, propolis comes from the hive in brown, waxy chunks.

HISTORICAL NOTES

Propolis has been used for time immemorial as both food and medicine. Many healers of antiquity knew of the medicinal qualities of propolis, including the Greeks who had three names for it. The ancients were not aware of everything propolis can do, but it has been used and appreciated for its antiseptic, anti-inflammatory, and infection-fighting properties for centuries. Propolis was extensively used during the Boer War as wound-dressing.

Throughout Europe, there are medical facilities known as apitherapy clinics. The term is derived from *Apis mellifera*, the Latin name for honeybees. Doctors in apitherapy clinics treat exclusively with bee pollen, propolis, and royal jelly, three of the products of the beehive. These clinics are especially popular in the countries of eastern Europe. Propolis is often called "Russian penicillin" because of the great amount of research the former USSR and its neighboring countries have conducted on this substance.

SCIENTIFIC FINDINGS

Extensive research around the world has confirmed that propolis has antibiotic, antiseptic, antibacterial, antifungal, antimicrobial, anti-inflammatory, and even antiviral properties. This is a very broad-spectrum medicinal that helps treat just about anything you can think of. Although most research on nature's medicine is conducted abroad, Columbia University is engaged in on-going research on an extract from propolis named CAPE (caffeic acid phenethyl ester). Results show that CAPE has very powerful antiviral properties.

TRADITIONAL USE

Internal. Simply sucking on a raw bit of propolis reputedly cures both infected teeth and sore throats amazingly quickly.

Abroad, country people often take their daily dose of preventive medicine by dropping a spoonful of homemade propolis tincture on a square of bread and eating it with their breakfast.

Health-food stores sell the tincture, as well as tablets and capsules, but not all stores carry raw chunks of propolis. Because of its waxy consistency, it's almost impossible to brew a tea from raw propolis. Instead, put a few drops of the tincture in any tea of your choice. That's much easier and tastes better, too. Propolis is very bitter. If you wish to make your own propolis tincture, please see Chapter 3 for preparation instructions.

External. Propolis cream is an excellent treatment for minor burns, cuts, or wounds of any kind. Propolis ointment or salve helps dry and heal pimples and pustules. It also helps prevent pits and scarring. Even adult acne succumbs to propolis. If you wish to make a propolis salve, please see Chapter 3.

CONSIDERATIONS

None of the sources I consulted listed any adverse reactions to the ingestion of propolis. An occasional case of nonspecific dermatitis has been tied to the substance's topical use, but such events are few and far between.

Psyllium *(Plantago psyllium)*

This herb is a well-known aid for the gastrointestinal tract. It is full of the dietary fiber that both treats and prevents constipation because it retains water, thereby softening the stools. Psyllium is helpful in warding off diverticulitis, colitis, and hemorrhoids. Because of the mucilage in it, psyllium lubricates and heals without irritating the mucous membranes of the intestines. It is the most popular mucilaginous herb in use today. Manufacturers of bulk laxatives and stool softeners (Metamucil, for example) use various forms of psyllium. Check out the ingredient labels sometime. Most of these preparations—and there are many, many of them—contain this herb.

DESCRIPTION AND PARTS USED

Psyllium is an annual, native to the Mediterranean regions of southern Europe, and to the Canary Islands, Northern Africa, and India. This tidy herb grows low to the ground and produces small white flowers. The parts used are the seeds, which are smooth ovals ranging from 1/16 to 1/8 inch long, and the thin, translucent hulls that encase the seeds.

HISTORICAL NOTES

Psyllium has been used for centuries, as a medicinal herb, as food, and as cattle fodder. Its name derives from the Greek word *psylla*, which translates to "flea." The ancients thought the seeds resembled those tiny creatures. In India, psyllium is used as a diuretic. In China, related species of this herb are used to treat bloody urine, coughing, and high blood pressure.

SCIENTIFIC FINDINGS

Those who lead sedentary lives have a need to stimulate the normal reflex activity of the bowel. Fiber-rich psyllium provides the necessary stimulation. It has been determined that psyllium works by increasing the volume of the intestinal contents. The mucilage in this herb swells when it comes into contact with water, softening the stool and stretching the intestines. As the walls of the intestine stretch to accommodate the increased bulk, peristaltic activity is initiated and increased in the bowel, and a comfortable movement ensues.

TRADITIONAL USE

Internal. Psyllium seeds are sold ground or powdered. Simply stir 1 teaspoon (1/6 ounce or 4 grams) of the herb into 1 cup of liquid and drink 2 to 3 times daily. The seeds—which are rich in fiber and mucilage and contain tannins—are the most powerful form of psyllium. You can also buy dried and powdered psyllium hulls. The hulls work more gently and do not contain tannin, which can cause irritation. If you are using the dried hulls, simply soak the recommended quantity overnight in a glass of warm water. The daily dose ranges from 1 1/4 to 2 1/2 teaspoons (1/5 to 1/3 ounce or 5 to 10 ten grams) taken 3 times a day.

CONSIDERATIONS

Every health authority on the planet agrees that those who eat a typical westernized diet low in fruits and vegetables and full of processed and manufactured foods need more fiber. Psyllium seeds can fill that need. However, it's necessary to start slowly and give your body time to get used to the increased fiber. Taking too much initially can cause gassiness and stomach discomfort. Given time, your body will adjust and the health benefits are great. Remember, the experts say drinking eight to ten glasses of water a day is important when adding fiber to the diet.

Red Clover *(Trifolium pratense)*

This sweet herb is an excellent overall tonic and blood purifier that fights infection and has relaxant and anti-inflammatory properties. It is, therefore, valuable in the treatment of irritated lungs, whooping cough, and many conditions where inflammation is a complication, including arthritis, gout, AIDS, and certain skin disorders. Red clover tea also works well as an appetite suppressant. It is traditionally used to help strengthen the system and restore vitality and energy. Because it is mild, red clover is even considered suitable for weak children.

DESCRIPTION AND PARTS USED

Red clover is a plant of the pastures. You've probably seen it when you were driving through the country. It is distinguished by its trefoil leaves and globes of small raspberry-red flowers. The whole plant has mild sedative properties, but it is the flower heads that are valued for their medicinal properties.

HISTORICAL NOTES

In one old herbal, red clover is described as being "God's greatest herbal blessing to mankind." The trinity of leaves joined at the stem was once considered evidence of the divine powers of this herb. That may be, but information about the historical uses of red clover is meager.

Native Americans used a weak tea of red clover to treat "sore eyes" and made a salve of it to treat burns. During the Industrial Revolution, red clover tea was the treatment of choice for "wasting diseases" such as rickets, tuberculosis, and cancer. One source revealed that the dried and ground blossoms of red clover were once smoked as an antiasthmatic treatment.

SCIENTIFIC FINDINGS

Red clover is not only a good medicinal, it qualifies as a good dietary supplement, too. Analysis shows this herb supplies vitamins A, B complex, C, F, and P. It contains choline, inositol, coumarins, glycosides, and a nice supply of minerals as well, including iron, selenium, cobalt, nickel, manganese, sodium, magnesium, calcium, and copper.

TRADITIONAL USE

Internal. To enjoy the tonic and blood-cleansing effects of red clover, follow the manufacturer's instructions regarding the amount of herb to use per cup and brew a strong tea. (For information on brewing tea, see Chapter 3.) Strain, add honey, and sip hot.

External. Red clover is said to cure even "old sores" when used as a wash or poultice. Please refer to Chapter 3 for directions on preparing these treatments.

CONSIDERATIONS

All sources seem to agree that red clover is both mild and safe.

Red Raspberry *(Rubus idaeus)*

Red raspberry is one of the traditional "woman's herbs." It is noted for its ability to ease uterine and intestinal spasms, and can help prevent hemorrhage. Because of its relaxing action, it quickly relieves menstrual cramps and can even ease hot flashes. Red raspberry tea helps strengthen the uterine wall, relieve labor pains, and ease childbirth. But it is not for women only.

Red raspberry is considered a reliable treatment for fevers, colds, and flu, as well as stomach problems, including nausea and diarrhea. Mild enough for children, it promotes healthy skin and nails, bones and teeth, and helps heal canker sores.

There are those who claim drinking raspberry leaf tea leads to a loss of weight. This herb is even sold as a reducing tea. Unfortunately, there is not one smidgen of evidence supporting the value of red raspberry as a reducing aid.

DESCRIPTION AND PARTS USED

The raspberry likes to grow near water and was originally a plant of the woodlands, although it is widely cultivated today. It is distinguished by leaves with silvery undersides. It has a thorny nature and puts forth small white flowers. The berries are brilliant red to winey-red, very juicy, and tart-sweet. Animals in the wild search out these plants and seem to enjoy munching on both the foliage and the fruits. The bark, leaves, and roots are the repositories of the medicinal properties.

HISTORICAL NOTES

In days gone by, pregnant women religiously took one cup of raspberry tea every day during the last two months of pregnancy to tone up their uterine muscles for labor and delivery. After the birth of the baby, one cup of raspberry tea was traditionally taken each day for several weeks more to help the uterus return to normal.

SCIENTIFIC FINDINGS

The old beliefs have been validated. Scientists have determined that this herb contains nutrients which act to strengthen the uterine wall. Raspberry does help relieve labor pains and promote an easier birth. In addition, it has been shown to reduce the incidence of false labor pains common to some mothers. Taking the tea after birth even acts to enrich the colostrum found in breast milk, which helps assure a newborn a healthy start in life.

Red raspberry contains vitamins A, some of the Bs, C, D, and E. It is rich in iron and calcium, and offers respectable amounts of phosphorus and manganese, as well as citric acid, pectin, and a bit of silicon.

TRADITIONAL USE

Internal. For a healing tea, pour 8 ounces of freshly boiled water over 7 1/4 teaspoons (1 ounce or 28.35 grams) of raspberry leaves. Cover and let the herb steep for 20 minutes. (For more information on brewing tea, see Chapter 3.)

CONSIDERATIONS

In spite of the fact that red raspberry tea eliminates morning sickness during pregnancy—and is often recommended for this use—women should not take the tea during the first seven months of pregnancy because this herb can relax the uterine wall. During the final two months of pregnancy, it is safe to take advantage of the strengthening and toning action red raspberry exerts on the uterus if your doctor gives the okay.

Rose Hips

You may already know that rose hips are very high in ascorbic acid. They are traditionally taken as an excellent natural source of vitamin C. But perhaps you don't know that this herb is a good blood purifer considered helpful against all infections, especially those affecting the bladder and kidneys. This herb also eases stress; battles coughs, colds, and flu; and is very nourishing to the skin.

DESCRIPTION AND PARTS USED

There are more different kinds of roses than of any other plant in the herb category, and they all provide rose hips. The rose family (*Rosaceae*) is composed of thorny shrubs native to Europe and North America. Rose hips are the fruits of members of this family. After the rose petals fall, the hips appear. These pods can be as small as a pea or as large as a marble, and they come in various colors. Although some are green, most hips are red or reddish-orange. The taste of rose hips is at once fruity and slightly spicy.

HISTORICAL NOTES

For a long time, rose hips were commonly used in cooking. Native Americans used rose hips as a food, and they were frequently stewed with sugar and spices. Sauce Saracen or Sarzyn was prepared by mixing rose hips with pounded almonds, cooking the mixture in wine, and adding sweetener.

SCIENTIFIC FINDINGS

Hard as it may be to believe, several varieties of rose hips are as much as sixty times richer in vitamin C than most oranges. Like most natural foods with a high content of vitamin C, rose hips also provide the bioflavonoids that make vitamin C work better.

The first serious investigation of the nutritive properties of rose hips was conducted during World War II when the beleagured countries of England, Sweden, and Norway were unable to get fresh citrus fruits. Knowing the importance of vitamin C to health, scientists began researching local botanicals, looking for a substitute. After testing many wild fruits and plants, the researchers discovered that rose hips were many times richer in this important vitamin than citrus fruits. The hips were promptly used in a variety of ways, including teas, soups, purees, puddings, jams, and jellies.

It has also been determined that rose hips provide B-complex, vitamins A, D, and E, are high in organic iron and calcium, and contain measurable amounts of potassium, sulphur, silica, and zinc, as well as fructose and tannins.

TRADITIONAL USE

Internal. To brew a healing tea of rose hips, use 1/2 to 1 teaspoon (1/12 to 1/6 ounce or 2 to 4 grams) of the dried and powdered fruit to 8 ounces of freshly boiled water. (For more information on brewing teas, see Chapter 3.) This tea has a mild fruit-tart taste. Stir in a spoonful of raw honey, if you wish.

CONSIDERATIONS

Consider rose hip tea a nutritive marvel of nature. No author I consulted had anything adverse to say about it.

Sage *(Salvia officinalis)*

Sage is said to refresh and stimulate the brain, relieve mental exhaustion, improve memory and the ability to concentrate. This herb has been credited with age-retarding and life-lengthening qualities for centuries.

An old Chinese adage says, "Sage for old age." In Chinese medicine, this herb is used to treat yin (cold) conditions such as a weakness of the stomach and digestive system. Sage is an excellent digestive aid with good carminative properties.

Because this herb helps slow excessive secretion of fluids, it is traditionally used to treat night sweats, abnormal perspiration, diarrhea, and dysentery. Sage is also a mild anti-inflammatory that is considered of value during the early stages of colds and flu, especially when nasal congestion is present. As a gargle, sage tea has been used for centuries against sore throat, canker sores, thrush, infected teeth, and gingivitis.

DESCRIPTION AND PARTS USED

Sage is a perennial plant that reaches about two feet in height. It likes a sheltered, partially sunny location and may need to be covered during severe winter weather. On its erect stems, sage bears small bluish flowers that are variegated with purple and white. The large leaves, which hold the medicinal properties, are a grayish-green and may be tinged with purple or red. Fresh sage has a pleasantly pungent scent.

HISTORICAL NOTES

Common garden sage has been revered for its healing qualities since the earliest times and is rich in historical lore. It was once considered the "savior" among all the healing herbs. Its botanical name, *Salvia*, comes from the Latin *salvere*, which means "to be saved." *Salvere* was shortened variously to sauja, then sauge, and finally, in Old English, to sawge, leading logically to sage, as we know this herb today.

This plant once enjoyed such a strong reputation as a longevity herb that learned physicians of the Middle Ages were heard to say, "Cur moriatur homo cui Salvia crescit in horto?" The translation reads, "Why should a man die whilst Sage grows in his garden?" A very old English proverb provides this assurance, "He that would live for aye, must eat Sage in May."

All the old herbals extol the virtues of sage. In his journal, Gerard wrote, "Sage is effective for quickening the senses and memory, strengthening the sinews and restoring health to those suffering from palsies of moist causes, removing shaking and trembling of the limbs."

The famed Culpeper himself wrote, "Sage provokes the urine and stayeth the bleeding of woundes and cleaneth ulcers and sores. The juice of Sage with Vinegar and honey put thereto is used to wash sore mouths and throats, as need requireth."

SCIENTIFIC FINDINGS

Sage is a natural antiseptic and is credited with other valuable properties as well. For example, a report published in Britain reads, in part, "Garden sage, a simple aromatic astringent, has recently undergone a series of tests. . . . Sage is a bactericide and fungicide of subtle and penetrating power. It scores a definite victory over penicillin-resistant substances and common oral pathogens. It is singularly helpful in oral thrush."

It's Not Just a Spice

You probably know sage mainly as a culinary herb. It's almost obligatory when preparing poultry. The following old "receipts"— both probably a century or so old—will give you a look at just two of the ways our ancestors used sage.

Rich Sage Tea

It is written that Rich Sage Tea is "a pleasant drink, cooling in fevers, and also a cleaner and purifier of the blood." We are also assured it is "highly serviceable as a stimulant in debility of the stomach and nervous system, and weakness of digestion generally."

From all accounts, a healing brew of Rich Sage Tea was a staple in many households of past centuries. Try it and see what you think.

1/2 ounce of fresh sage leaves
1 ounce fine sugar
1/4 ounce grated rind of lemon
juice from the same lemon
1 quart boiled water

1. *Assemble the first four ingredients in a container with a cover. Pour the freshly boiled water over the assembled ingredients.*
2. *Cover and permit the tea to steep for 30 minutes. Strain and bottle for future use.*

Directions for Use

Take one wineglassful as needed.

Candied Sage Leaves

I do believe Candied Sage Leaves may have been the forerunner of the after-dinner mint. This very old use of sage makes sense when you remember that this herb is a good digestive aid with carminative properties.

1 handful fresh well-formed sage leaves (two leaves per person)
1 egg white
1 tablespoon water
fine sugar

1. *Wash the leaves gently and set aside to dry thoroughly.*
2. *Add the water to the egg white and beat until frothy.*
3. *Dip the leaves quickly into the beaten egg white.*
4. *While the leaves are still wet, sift fine sugar over them until they are lightly coated and let dry thoroughly.*

Directions for Use

Serve two Candied Sage Leaves to each dinner guest.

Of perhaps more interest is the fact that this herb has been found to act beneficially on the cortex of the brain. It apparently really can be an aid to concentration and improving memory.

TRADITIONAL USE

Internal. Sage tea requires longer steeping than most other herbs. Pour 8 ounces of freshly boiled water over 1 3/4 teaspoons (1/4 ounce or 7.08 grams) of sage leaves. Cover and allow the tea to steep for 10 minutes. Strain and sip hot. (For more information on brewing tea, see Chapter 3.) Sage tea is useful as a gargle for a sore throat. To help heal ulcerations of the mouth, just swish a mouthful around the affected area several times daily.

External. A sage poultice is considered valuable for nasal congestion and in all serious cases involving the throat and chest. The recommendation is to sip sage tea while the aromatic poultice works double-time to relieve infection and congestion. (For directions on preparing a poultice, see Chapter 3.)

If you're out in the garden and get stung by a bee or nipped by any other little creature, crush a sage leaf and rub it on the spot. The risk of infection will be lessened and the hurt and itch will be relieved quickly.

CONSIDERATIONS

Sage tea may be taken up to three times daily, but treatment should not exceed one week.

Sarsaparilla *(Smilax officinalis)*

Sarsaparilla is a tonic and blood purifier with the ability to favorably tone up the whole system. It also successfully treats psoriasis, eczema, and other skin diseases. As a historic depurative, sarsaparilla is traditionally used against disorders arising from blood impurities, such as arthritis, rheumatism, gout, and digestive disorders, including ulcerative colitis. This herb helps fight certain venereal diseases, including syphilis and herpes, reduces stress on the liver, is an effective fever reducer, and has mild antibiotic properties.

DESCRIPTION AND PARTS USED

Smilax officinalis is at home in tropical climes, including South America. It has a long slender root with short, thick rhizomes. This plant produces a vine that both trails on the ground and climbs hospitable trees by means of tiny tendrils that emerge from its evergreen leaves. The root flavors the soft drink of the same name and is the part of the plant used for medicinal purposes.

HISTORICAL NOTES

During the sixteenth century, sarsaparilla was the European drug of choice for the treatment of syphilis. Many believed syphilis came to Europe from the West Indies with Columbus' sailors. At this time, medical men thought it logical that the cure would originate in the same region as the disease. The hope that sarsaparilla was a cure for syphilis was so great that the herb was imported at large expense from the Caribbean and South America. Before that time, the venereal disease had been treated with mercury, a "cure" that often caused more deaths than the disease. "At least," so stated a doctor of the times, "the patient on mercury mercifully died sooner." Syphilis drove men mad and presaged an agonizing death.

Chinese physicians, who keep meticulous records, have long used sarsaparilla to treat syphilis. According to their clinical observations, sarsaparilla is effective in about 90 percent of acute cases, and 50 percent of chronic cases.

Sarsaparilla was growing wild long before the colonists arrived on these shores. Native Americans used it, and the settlers embraced it quickly. An early American herbal had this to say: "Sarsaparilla is deservedly esteemed for its medicinal virtues, being a gentle sudorific, and very powerful in attenuating the blood when impeded by gross humours. The bark of the roots, which alone should be used in medicine, is of a bitterish flavor, but aromatic."

As the demand for sarsaparilla grew, patent medicines claiming to contain this herb sold like wildfire. One angry doctor wrote, "Such is the furor for swallowing it, that the manufacturers employ steam engines in its preparation and these syrups and extracts of sarsaparilla are becoming the chief exports of the commercial emporiums. Soon, enough quantity will be made to supply all creation with physics for a century to come."

In 1911, nine "sarsaparilla" patent medicines were analyzed by scientists working under the auspices of the Connecticut government. They found these formulas contained mostly other herbs, including yellow dock, burdock, sassafras, poke root, wintergreen, licorice, senna, black cohosh, prickly ash, mandrake, and a variety of other botanicals and chemicals, with just a smidgin of sarsaparilla. Shortly after this deception was discovered, sarsaparilla was taken off the official drug plant list, although it had long been officially accepted as a stimulant, alterative, and diaphoretic.

SCIENTIFIC FINDINGS

There is evidence showing that sarsaparilla is a possible endotoxin binder. Endotoxins are constituents of bacteria that are absorbed by the body. The liver has the responsibility for filtering out these harmful compounds before they enter the bloodstream. However, if the liver falls down on the job, or if there are just too many endotoxins, they can spill over into the blood. The result is the type of inflammation and cell damage that occurs in such diseases as ulcerative colitis, gout, arthritis, and psoriasis. Absorbed endotoxins also produce fever. Sarsaparilla binds with endotoxins, helping the liver detoxify the blood.

Science has validated the use of sarsaparilla against diseases that are aggravated by endotoxins. For example, individuals suffering from psoriasis have been shown to have high levels of endotoxins in their blood. A clinical study of psoriasis patients found that an extract of sarsaparilla greatly improved symptoms in 62 percent of the patients. Even better, 18 percent of those so treated were completely relieved of the disease.

However, those who believe in sarsaparilla's much-touted reputation as either a muscle-builder or sexual rejuvenator are doomed to disappointment. The steroid-like substances in this herb are not absorbed by the body. There's no testosterone in it either. Sarsaparilla does contain a compound that can be converted to testosterone in a laboratory, but this reaction does not take place within the human body.

TRADITIONAL USE

Internal. Sarsaparilla tea is brewed as a decoction of 1/4 to 1 teaspoon (.034 to .137 ounces or 1 to 4 grams) of the root, and may be taken 3 times daily. (For more information on preparing a decoction, see Chapter 3.)

CONSIDERATIONS

No adverse effects from the use of sarsaparilla tea have been reported. Nonetheless, the experts caution against taking large doses over a long period of time.

Sassafras *(Sassafras officinale)*

Sassafras can no longer be recommended as a safe botanical. It is included here only for its historical interest. This uniquely American herb was once considered an important ingredient in traditional spring tonics and, like sarsaparilla, it was considered valuable as a treatment for syphilis. This flavorful and aromatic herb has also been used to mask the taste of less palatable botanicals. The oil was used as a rubefacient in the treatment of arthritis and rheumatism.

DESCRIPTION AND PARTS USED

The sassafras tree is indigenous to the Americas, where it is found all along the eastern coastline. It can attain a great height in the south, where the tree may grow as tall as 100 feet. Northern climes are not as hospitable, however. In chilly climates, this herb develops into nothing more than a straggly shrub. Tree or bush, sassafras puts forth many slender branches with "mitten-shaped" three-lobed leaves. The flowers are intensely fragrant. The bark, which is the part used, is smooth and orangish-brown.

HISTORICAL NOTES

One of the legends concerning sassafras was immortalized in the writings of one G.B. Emerson in his book *Trees and Shrubs of Massachusetts*, published in 1894. Emerson wrote, "This tree has the credit of having aided in the discovery of America, as it is said to have been its strong fragrance, smelt by Columbus, which encouraged him to persevere, and enabled him to convince his mutinous crew that land was near." Whether the tale is true or not, historians agree that Spanish explorers came upon sassafras in Florida, learned of its uses from the Native Americans, and subsequently popularized the herb throughout Europe.

There are many references to sassafras in the writings of those who recorded the medicinal practices of Native Americans. For example, an early article in the *Smithsonian Report*, carried this information: "Seneca warriors carried the powdered leaves, women employed it as tonic after childbirth, it was used in cases of rheumatism, and as a diuretic; and drinking Sassafras tea as a spring tonic was so much a part of life on the American frontier that the Iroquois herbalists regularly peddled the root bark on the doorsteps of their white neighbors."

In 1804, a Dr. Barton of Philadelphia wrote an essay expressing his doubts about the wholesale use of this herb. He wrote, "The oil of Sassafras, when externally applied to the body in rheumatic afflictions is remarkable for its power of shifting the pain from its original seat, but not always to the advantage of the patient. I believe, however, that it is a medicine well adapted to many cases of rheumatism in its chronic stage, though even here it may prove injurious."

Sassafras was listed as an acceptable aromatic, diaphoretic, antiseptic, and rubefacient drug and ant repellent in the *United States Pharmacopoeia* from 1840 to 1910.

SCIENTIFIC FINDINGS

Sassafras oil and safrole, both major constituents of the volatile oils found in sassafras root bark, were once the flavoring of choice for root beer. In fact, that's how root beer got its name. But these ingredients have been banned for use in root beer for close to fifty years. It is now known that safrole inhibits the action of important liver enzymes. Even worse, scientists have determined that sassafras causes cancer in rats when taken in large amounts.

CONSIDERATIONS

If you had your mind set on sassafras tea for some reason, reset it. I don't care what great-grandmother believed. This time, she was wrong. Don't sweat it. Just refer to the Trouble-Shooting Guide on page 92 and make another selection.

Saw Palmetto *(Serenoa repens)*

Saw palmetto gained a reputation as an aphrodisiac because it is traditionally used to improve the functioning of the reproductive glands, both male and female. It is also used to soothe sexual organs irritated by intense sexual activity, a condition sometimes smilingly called "honeymoon cystitis."

In males, saw palmetto has proven valuable in the treatment of noncancerous prostate enlargement. This herb can even help relieve the need for frequent urination at night when the cause is pressure against the bladder. It can stimulate testicular function as well.

DESCRIPTION AND PARTS USED

The saw palmetto is a small palm tree. It's not one of those skyscraper palms. The mature tree reaches a height of from six to ten feet. It has the same type of large leaves that crown the tops of most palms. Saw palmetto is indigenous to the Atlantic coastline of North America, but it likes a comfortable climate. Its habitat extends along the coast from South Carolina to Florida. The inch-long oval berries, which run from deep reddish-brown to almost black, hold the medicinal components.

HISTORICAL NOTES

This herb has long had a reputation as an aphrodisiac and was considered a potent tonic for the reproductive glands. Native Americans were making use of saw palmetto berries in cases of genitourinary disturbances, including tired testes, long before the colonists arrived and adopted it. It was also used to treat women with disorders of the mammary glands.

Saw palmetto is not officially recognized in the United States. However, the herb is so well accepted in Germany as treatment for benign prostate enlargement that it is sold over-the-counter for that purpose.

SCIENTIFIC FINDINGS

Studies confirm that more than 50 percent of males between the ages of forty and sixty have benign prostatic hypertrophy (BPH). This medical term translates to enlargement of the prostate gland. BPH can be caused by an accumulation of testosterone, which the prostate promptly converts to dihydrotestosterone (DHT). DHT causes the cells to multiply like wildfire and the gland enlarges to accommodate the growing number of cells. This condition gives rise to some annoying symptoms, including a need to urinate frequently day and night, and the inability to fully empty the bladder because the stream becomes feeble. Left untreated, the bladder outlet will eventually close completely. Surgery is often necessary.

However, an extract of saw palmetto berries has shown an amazing ability to benefit this condition. The extract prevents testosterone from being converted to DHT and actually inhibits its binding to the cells, which further increases the breakdown and natural excretion of DHT. In a double-blind study of men suffering from BPH, 160 mg of the extract twice daily racked up some impressive clinical results. In subjects treated with it, nighttime urination decreased by close to 50 percent; flow rate increased by over 50 percent; and the residual urine left in the bladder decreased 42 percent. None of the men receiving the placebo reported improvement. Other studies of this substance have tallied up similar success rates.

One scientific article reports that saw palmetto berries may be useful as treatment for hirsutism (heavy growth of hair) and androgen (steroid hormones responsible for masculine characteristics) excess in women. If you are a woman with unwanted male characteristics, including male-pattern hair growth, you may wish to investigate this herb further.

TRADITIONAL USE

Internal. To brew a healing saw palmetto tea, add 1 heaping teaspoon (1/6 ounce or 4 grams) of the dried berries to 8 ounces of boiling water. (For more on brewing tea, see Chapter 3.) To obtain a therapeutic dose—one equivalent to 160 mg of the extract—take 2 1/2 teaspoons (1/3 ounce or 10 grams) of the tea twice daily.

CONSIDERATIONS

I am happy to tell you that saw palmetto has no significant toxic side effects. None have been reported with the extract; none have been reported with the tea.

Skullcap *(Scutellaria lateriflora)*

Skullcap is a champion nervine, calmative, and antispasmodic. It is the herbal remedy of choice for all nervous disorders, including stress, tics, insomnia, and hysteria, as well as central nervous system disorders, such as convulsions, delirium tremens (DTs), and St. Vitus dance. This herb is also considered valuable in the treatment of nervous headaches, neuralgia, muscle spasms, and muscle cramps.

DESCRIPTION AND PARTS USED

Varieties of skullcap are found all over the world. The French name for skullcap is *toque*, which describes a brimless close-fitting cap. The hooded flowers of this plant do indeed resemble a close-fitting cap that hugs the skull.

Skullcap makes itself at home in just about any type soil, but it prefers a damp and sunny, open location where it can spread out. This plant has short-stalked leaves and grows anywhere from six inches to eighteen inches high. It flowers in June and bears hooded blue flowers in rows along its branching stems. Everything growing above ground is used medicinally.

HISTORICAL NOTES

Both the herb's generic and botanical names come from the Latin *scutella*, from which the English word "skull" derives. The "cap" of a skull is the rounded upper portion that protects the brain, thus skullcap. Think of a "beanie," if you prefer, although "beanie" doesn't make it as a name for an herb.

In the past, skullcap has been used against epilepsy and hydrophobia with varying degrees of success. It was once known as "mad dog weed." One old herbal says skullcap "soothes excessive sexual desires." Another says this herb is a "sure remedy for the explosive headaches suffered by school teachers who have a frequent need to urinate."

SCIENTIFIC FINDINGS

Skullcap contains a moderate amount of zinc and trace amounts of some minerals, as well as vitamins A, C and E, plus tannins, sugars, volatile oils, fats, flavonoids, and a glycoside. It has been determined that the herb has mild antibacterial properties, but little research has centered on skullcap. Its reputation as a sedative and antispasmodic rests mostly on anecdotal evidence, but it seems clear that these properties exist.

TRADITIONAL USE

Internal. When taken as tea, this potent herb is brewed using 7 1/4 teaspoons (1 ounce or 28.35 grams) of the powdered herb to twelve ounces of freshly boiled water. (For more information on brewing teas, see Chapter 3.) Take a half-cupful (4 ounces) every 4 hours. Do not exceed 3 half-cupfuls (twelve ounces total) of skullcap tea in any 24-hour period. Add a drizzle of honey to the tea, if you like.

CONSIDERATIONS

Do not exceed the recommended dosage. An overdose of skullcap can cause giddiness, stupor, confusion, twitchings of the limbs, and irregular pulse. Skullcap is immensely useful and has been known to work when nothing else helps, but it is definitely for occasional use only.

Spearmint *(Mentha spicata)*

Spearmint has been valued for centuries as an excellent digestive. It stimulates the salivary glands, increases gastric secretions, and eases indigestion and gas pains. It is gentle and effective when applied against nausea and vomiting, and is even safe for children. This herb is also traditionally used to treat colds, flu, chills, and dizziness.

DESCRIPTION AND PARTS USED

Spearmint can attain a height of almost three feet. Its tall erect stems are without branches, but each stem puts forth many smooth, bright green leaves that have unevenly toothed edges. Spearmint bears flowers in midsummer on a single flower stalk. The blossoms vary in color from almost white to a deep purple. The leaves and the oil they contain make spearmint a valuable herb.

HISTORICAL NOTES

Spearmint is native to the Mediterranean countries and has been valued since ancient times. The Romans carried spearmint to what is now England. Everywhere this fragrant herb was introduced, people began to cultivate it. Spearmint is mentioned in all the early medieval lists of plants, and convent gardens of the ninth century featured the herb. Indeed, Chaucer described such a garden as containing "a little path of mintes full and fenill greene." History records that spearmint was one of the plants brought from England to the Americas by the Pilgrim fathers.

Many old writings extol spearmint as an aid to digestion. For example, in his *Materia Medica*, Gerard wrote, "It will not suffer milke to cruddle [curdle] in the stomacke, and therefore it is put in milke that is drunke, lest those that drinke therof should be strangled." In *Garden of Pleasure*, Parkinson wrote, "Spere Mynte should be outwardly applied or inwardly drunke to strengthen and comforte weak stomackes."

SCIENTIFIC FINDINGS

Spearmint is a good source of vitamins A and C, and a minor source of B complex, calcium, sulphur, iron, iodine, magnesium, and potassium. The chief constituent of its volatile oil is carvone, but the esters of acetic, butyric and caproic or caprylic acids are the constituents that are responsible for the distinctive scent and flavor of spearmint.

Oil of spearmint is expressed from the fresh plant. The shoots are taken in August, just as the plant begins to flower. It takes 350 pounds of spearmint leaves to produce a single pound of oil.

TRADITIONAL USE

Internal. Spearmint tea is made by pouring 8 ounces of freshly boiled water over 1 level tablespoonful (1/2 ounce or 12 grams)

The Sleeping Potion Pillow

Aromatherapy is yet another way to use spearmint. Master herbalist Culpeper wrote, "Being smelled unto, Spere Mynte is comfortable for the hede and memory . . . Rose leaves and Mynte, applied outwardly, bring reste, repose, and sleep." In Germany, aromatherapy pillows are called "Krauterkissen," which translates to "herb cushion." Many European specialty shops offer delightful herb cushions filled with various deliciously fragrant herb and flower blends. The following are very old directions for stitching an herbal pillow that can lull you pleasantly to sleep:

Filling:
3 cups dried spearmint leaves
3 cups dried rose leaves
1 cup dried and powdered cloves
1 ounce orris root*

Covering:
2 squares of tightly woven fabric (12 to 14 inches),
ticking or chintz
thread

1. *Crush the spearmint and rose leaves well. (If you want to follow tradition, use a mortar and pestle. I find it easier to put a quantity of leaves into a zip-lock plastic bag and crush them using a rolling pin or heavy glass.)*

2. *Put the crushed leaves into a bowl, add the cloves, and mix well.*

3. *Sprinkle the orris root over all and blend it in thoroughly. Orris root is the fixative; don't leave it out.*

4. *Place 1 square of fabric on top of the other, wrong sides facing out, with the 4 corners aligned. Stitch tightly around all 4 sides, leaving about a 3-inch opening on one side for inserting the herbs. Turn right side out.*

5. *Once you have put in the crushed herbs, turn the raw edges under and stitch up the opening.*

*Orris root is a fixative, a substance used to set and hold in the fragrance of herbs. It comes from the florentine iris, the root of which is carefully dried and stored for at least two years before being ground into a fine powder.

Directions for Use

Old herbals say this aromatic herbal pillow will overcome melancholia, bring sleep, and ensure sweet dreams. Just tuck this loosely-stuffed soft and "cushy" pillow under your cheek and drift off to dreamland.

---

of the dried leaves. Cover, allow to steep for 3 minutes, strain, add a spoonful of honey, and enjoy. (For more information on brewing teas, see Chapter 3.)

If you wish to follow a pleasant, very old Continental custom, put a saucer of powdered dried spearmint on the dinner table and invite your guests to dust some on a bowl of pea soup, or sprinkle some on a sauce or gravy.

External. Crushed fresh spearmint leaves can take the hurt out of insect bites, including bee or wasp stings. Just grab a couple and scrub the spot. An old herbal says that washing a "scurfy head" (one with dandruff) with a concoction composed of spearmint leaves crushed in vinegar will effect a cure.

CONSIDERATIONS

Members of the mint family are completely free of toxic side effects. Spearmint is no exception.

St. John's Wort
(*Hypericum perforatum*)

This ancient herb is useful against bronchitis and lung congestion arising from any cause. It is considered very helpful for expelling heavy phlegm from the chest or lungs. St. John's wort is used to treat people with suppressed urination and, although it seems contradictory, it is used to stem bed-wetting. The herb has traditionally been used to ease painful menstruation, soothe the pangs of afterbirth, and treat many menopausal symptoms.

St. John's wort is one of the herbs traditionally prescribed for jangled nerves and melancholia. The tea is especially helpful in cases of neuralgia and/or headaches, especially if they are accompanied by nervousness or excitability verging on hysteria, or occur during depression. Headaches with symptoms such as throbbing on the top of the head or a heavy lethargic feeling in the head are often eased by St. John's wort.

Used externally, this herb is said to bring down swellings and heal old wounds, even festering wounds, when nothing else seems to help. It also helps bring boils to a head, and cleanses abscesses, neglected cuts, and bad insect stings.

DESCRIPTION AND PARTS USED

St. John's wort grows on sunny hillsides, on dry pastureland, and at the edges of woods and roads; it isn't fussy about its environment. A perennial that grows to a height of one to three feet, the plant has an unusual angular stalk that puts forth perforated leaves. The flowers branch out at the tip of the stems. If you crush these golden yellow flowers, you'll end up with a bright red stain on your fingers. The red "dye" comes from the small dark points inside the calyx and on the tips of the petals. Traditionally, the whole plant is used medicinally; however, the FDA approves only the leaves for internal use.

HISTORICAL NOTES

St. John's wort was brought to the United States from Europe early in American history. Long believed magical and mystical, the herb was used in ceremonies of exorcism designed to drive away demons. It was once called *Fuga daemonum*, which translates to "scare devil." The generic name *Hypericum* comes from the Greek—*hyper* meaning "over" and *ereike* meaning "hearth"—because the herb grows in sandy soil. *Perforatum* refers to the small dots in the leaves that look like holes or perforations, but which are actually subsurface oil glands.

Most Christian legends link this herb to John the Baptist. In medieval times, maidens wore garlands of the plant as they danced

St. John's Wort Oil

It is written that St. John's wort oil is the cure for many skin conditions, including sores that refuse to heal, old wounds, boils, abscesses, nasty cuts, bites and stings, and on and on. This oil is an ancient time-tested remedy that's nice to have ready against future need. Here's a very old "receipt" for preparing this herbal oil. You'll notice that the directions differ from the general instructions given in Chapter 3.

*1 fresh plant full of just-bloomed flowers
1 cup pure water (bottled or spring water)
18 ounces virgin olive oil*

1. *Crush a quantity of the fresh flowers well, measuring as you go. (A mortar and pestle may sound old fashioned, but it's the easiest way. If you don't have one of these gadgets handy, use the back of a large spoon.) You need to end up with 3/4 cup of crushed flowers.*

2. *Put the pure water into a medium-sized bowl and stir in the crushed flowers. Add the olive oil and blend as best you can.*

3. *Pour the mixture into a wide-necked glass jar of sufficient size to allow the mixture to double in volume. Leave the jar uncovered and put it in a warm place to ferment. Stir daily. (Tiny gasseous bubbles will form and the mixture will increase in volume. Fermentation will occur in 3 to 5 days.) When the mixture has almost doubled in size and is a mass of airy bubbles, stir down one more time.*

4. *Cap the jar so it is airtight and let the oil rest in a dark place away from sunlight for about 6 weeks, or until the contents have turned a luminous red. Pour off the oil, which will have risen to the top, leaving the watery layer of flowers behind. Discard the flowers.*

5. *Put the oil into a bottle with an airtight lid. The oil is now ready to be used both internally and externally.*

Directions for Use

Take 1 teaspoonful 2 to 3 times per day to calm a nervous stomach or stimulate a lazy gallbladder. If using the oil to treat depression, be aware that the benefits will not be apparent for 2 to 3 weeks.

Rub into the skin to relieve the pain of rheumatism and lumbago. Soak a clean cotton cloth in the oil and bind it around the affected area to ease sprains and strained muscles.

---

around bonfires in celebration of St. John's birthday. The bright red oil contained in the leaves of St. John's wort has been likened to both the blood and wounds of Jesus Christ, as well as to St. John the Baptist's blood. Country folk sometimes called the red stain left on their hands "Mary's sweat." No matter which interpretation you prefer, the religious connection is clear.

SCIENTIFIC FINDINGS

The mood-altering effects of St. John's wort have been substantiated. A clinical study of fifteen patients suffering from clinical depression showed that this herb can relieve the symptoms of anxiety, depression, and feelings of worthlessness that often accompany the condition. It also relieved both insomnia and hypersomnia (a need for excessive sleep).

In an initial study, scientists at the New York University Medical Center and the Weizmann Institute of Science in Israel showed that an extract of the herb can inhibit some viruses, including HIV (human immunodeficiency virus), which is associated with AIDS (acquired immune deficiency syndrome). The scientists caution against excessive optimism. Just because mice responded positively doesn't mean people will. The scientists point to the need for much more study before St. John's wort can be recommended as an adjunctive treatment for AIDS patients.

TRADITIONAL USE

Internal. St. John's wort is a rough and tough herb that is brewed by decoction. (For more information on preparing decoctions, see

Chapter 3.) To make a healing tea, pour 8 ounces of water over 1 heaping teaspoonful (2/5 ounce or 12 grams) of the dried herb. Simmer for 3 minutes. Strain. Use sparingly. No dosage has been established for St. John's wort.

External. For a quick-fix wash, brew an extra-strong tea, strain, cool, and apply as needed. (For more information, see Chapter 3.)

CONSIDERATIONS

Because this herb exerts a powerful antidepressant effect on its own, it should not be taken with any other antidepressant. It interacts unfavorably with L-dopa and tryptophan, and should not be taken with foods containing tyramine, such as cheese, beer, wine, herring, and yeast. It increases photosensitivity, thereby increasing the risk of sunburn, rashes, and irregular pigmentation. Anyone who spends a lot of time outdoors should select another herb.

Uva Ursi *(Arctostaphylos uva ursi)*

Uva ursi, pronounced yuva ursee, is traditionally prescribed for kidney and bladder infections, especially when water retention is a problem. This bitter herb has long been used successfully in the treatment of inflammatory diseases of the urinary tract, including urethritis and cystitis, and is said to help dissolve kidney stones. It is considered valuable against disorders of the spleen, liver, pancreas, and small intestines.

DESCRIPTION AND PARTS USED

A small evergreen shrub, uva ursi is found throughout Europe and in the northern United States. This shrub grows sideways and can eventually spread into a low-growing bushy clump that covers an area up to fifteen feet. It makes quite a nice ground cover. Uva ursi has a long, tough root that sends out burrowing stems which turn upward and attain a height of from four to six inches. Its flowers can be pink or white; the fruit can be bright red or pink. The leaves, which contain this herb's medicinal properties, are only 1/2 to 1 inch long.

HISTORICAL NOTES

Uva ursi means "the bear's grape" in Latin, which explains why the herb is also known as bear berry. Evidence shows that this herb was highly valued by the celebrated Welsh "Physicians of Myddfai" as far back as the 13th century. Uva ursi first appeared in the *London Pharmacopoeia* in 1788, but it was in common use throughout Europe for hundreds of years before it was officially recognized.

Native Americans called this plant *Kinnikinnick* and ranked it right up there with acorns as nutritious food. The leaves were used for smoking. The berries were variously eaten raw, juiced and fermented into cider, ground and cooked as porridge, or made into jelly.

SCIENTIFIC FINDINGS

Scientific investigation of this herb has centered on extracted arbutin, the most active constituent of uva ursi. It totals from 7 to 9 percent of the components found in the leaves. Research shows that arbutin has marked antiseptic and diuretic action. To do its duty, arbutin must be converted to hydroquinone in the urinary tract. However, when extracted arbutin is administered, bacteria in the intestines break it down before it can be absorbed, which destroys its usefulness. When the whole herb is administered, bacterial breakdown of arbutin does not occur. Components in the herb prevent the breakdown of the helpful arbutin and more is converted to hydroquinone. There's yet another benefit of using the whole herb. Full antibiotic activity of the arbutin depends on the alkalinity of the urine, and other constituents of the herb help increase the alkalinity of urine.

TRADITIONAL USE

Internal. To brew a healing uva ursi tea, pour 8 ounces of freshly boiled water over 1 3/4 teaspoons (1/4 ounce or 7.08 grams) of the dried leaves. Cover, steep for 5 minutes, strain, and sip hot. The traditional dose is 1 cup of tea taken 3 times daily. (For more information on brewing teas, please see Chapter 3.)

CONSIDERATIONS

Hydroquinone has been shown to be toxic at 1 gram. Toxicity, of course, depends on how much arbutin is actually converted into hydroquinone in the urinary tract and there's no way to predict that. Symptoms range from nausea and vomiting to convulsions and collapse. Do not exceed the recommended dose.

paedia, master herbalist Potter says, "Valerian allays pain and promotes sleep. It is strongly nervine without any narcotic effects. The infusion of one ounce to one pint of boiling water should be taken in wineglassful doses."

This ancient herb has been called the "valium of the nineteenth century." It was once widely prescribed in Europe to treat anxiety, nervous tension, and even panic attacks.

SCIENTIFIC FINDINGS

Recent studies have shown that valerian has a soothing effect on the entire central nervous system. Even when a person is extremely agitated, a cup of valerian tea can relieve that "hyper" feeling with its calming effects. However, the primary use for valerian is the same today as it was yesterday: This herb is nature's first choice as a sleep inducer.

In a double-blind study of 128 subjects, those given valerian extract fell asleep sooner, slept better, and awoke without the "drugged-out hangover" feeling that is an unwanted side effect of many over-the-counter sleep remedies. A later study confirmed these effects. It was also determined that valerian is just as effective as small doses of barbiturates and benzodiazepines. But the man-made chemical compounds leave the user feeling drugged in the morning, while the herbal remedy does not.

TRADITIONAL USE

Internal. To prepare valerian tea, it's necessary to make a cold infusion. Valerian is sensitive to heat and important healing properties may be lost if this herb is brewed with boiling water. Pour 8 ounces of cold water over 1 level teaspoon (1/6 ounce or 4 grams) of chopped valerian root. Cover and let the herb infuse overnight. Take 2 to 3 cups of tea per day, warmed to sipping temperature if you wish. (For more information on making cold infusions, see Chapter 3.)

To treat insomnia, drink 1 cup of valerian tea 30 to 45 minutes before going to bed. If a single cup of tea doesn't do the trick, the experts say to take a look at other factors that contribute to insomnia, such as an intake of caffeine too close to bedtime. On the other hand, if you sleep solidly after 1 cup but find yourself still sleepy when the alarm goes off in the morning, reduce the dosage.

External. A valerian bath is an old Victorian remedy for nervous upsets. Because of its pleasant smell, a valerian bath qualifies as aromatherapy as well. If you wish to enjoy a leisurely and soothing soak, please see Chapter 3 for directions on preparing an herbal bath.

CONSIDERATIONS

Valerian is a safe and effective sleep-promoting aid. Even the FDA approves of it. It has the label GRAS (generally regarded as safe), meaning this herb has been approved for food use.

White Willow *(Salix alba)*

White willow bark tea has been used down through the ages as a fever-reducer, pain-reliever, and anti-inflammatory agent. This herb breaks fevers, eases headaches, and reduces the pain and swelling of affected joints and sore, aching muscles. Because it works on the central nervous system as well as the musculoskeletal system, willow tea can ease stress and tension, both mental and physical.

DESCRIPTION AND PARTS USED

The graceful willow thrives in moist, even wet, locations and loves the banks of rivers, streams, and lakes. Because of their extensive root systems, willow trees are able to anchor and hold the land against shore-line erosion. The willow is indigenous to Europe, but has been well naturalized in North America. The active properties of this historic medicinal rest in its bark.

HISTORICAL NOTES

The family name of the willow—*Salix*—refers to its affinity for wet places. It comes from the Celtic *sal*, meaning "near," and *lis* meaning "water." This ancient herb turns up frequently through-out recorded history. For example, willow prescriptions can be found on a 4,000-year-old Sumerian tablet; Egyptian papyri dating from the sixteenth century B.C. extol the uses of willow, as do very old Assyrian tablets. The famed Greek physician Dioscorides described its uses centuries ago. Galen, another Greek physician, used willow bark to treat inflammations, and Hippocrates pre-scribed willow bark tea to treat pain and fever.

Native Americans were also well acquainted with the remedial powers of the willows. The bark, brewed into tea, was used for many purposes. The Natchez, Creeks, Alabamas and other tribes decocted the bark and both drank the tea and bathed in it to reduce fever and ease headaches and painful rheumatic joints. California tribes used decocted brews to treat lumbago and head-aches, and other Western Indians drank the tea to induce sweating to break a fever and treat a cold.

In the eighteenth century, one Reverend Stone learned of the success medicine men were having treating rheumatism with willow bark tea. He promptly brewed his own decoctions, tried the remedy on settlers who suffered from rheumatism, and confirmed that the tea effectively relieved pain.

SCIENTIFIC FINDINGS

In 1827, a French chemist named Leroux extracted the active substance in willow bark that provides its pain-relieving proper-ties. He named it "salicin," derived from *Salix*. Salicin is the source of salicylic acid, which you probably recognize as kissing-kin to aspirin.

During the late 1800s, chemists all over the world tried to develop a synthetic version of salicylic acid. A young chemist who worked for Farbenfabriken Bayer Aktiengegesellschaft, Leverkusen, of Cologne, Germany, won the race. He tested an acetyl ester of salicylic acid on his arthritic father, found it was effective, and acetylsalicylic acid, better known as aspirin, was born. For a very long time, most of us thought "Bayer" was aspirin's first name. Nonetheless, in spite of the successful synthesis, salicin was listed in the *United States Pharmacopoeia* from 1882 through 1926. It was still considered an official medicine in the 1950 edition of the *United States Dispensatory*, and was listed as such in the *National Formulary* as late as 1955. Salicin's use as an official medicinal came to an end when mass production of acetylsalicylic acid brought production costs down and profit margins up.

TRADITIONAL USE

Internal. To make willow bark tea, you must prepare a decoction. Put 4 tablespoons plus 2 teaspoons (2 ounces or 56.7 grams) of dried and flaked bark in a pot with 16 ounces of water. Cover the pot, simmer for 6 minutes, and strain. Take 1 cupful of the tea 3 times daily. (For more information on preparing decoctions, see Chapter 3.)

External. With apologies to the Native Americans who bathed in willow water to relieve painful joints and aching muscles, this medicinal seems to work better from the inside out than from the outside in.

CONSIDERATIONS

White willow bark tea has the same properties—and the same potential to irritate the gastrointestinal lining—as aspirin.

Wintergreen *(Gaultheria procumbens)*

This hot herb, a noted stimulant traditionally taken in small doses, acts on the stomach, heart, and respiratory system. Wintergreen is considered valuable against rheumatic pain, joint pain, lumbago, gout, sciatica, headache, and sore, aching muscles. There's a use for wintergreen from top to bottom: Gargling with the tea relieves a sore and inflammed throat; douching with the tea helps get rid of a yeast infection.

It was once thought that an application of the oil expressed from the leaves could eliminate warts, corns, callouses, cysts, and even tattoos. A poultice *can* help bring down swellings and boils.

DESCRIPTION AND PARTS USED

Wintergreen is a small evergreen shrub that feels at home in woodlands and clearings from Canada to Georgia. It hugs the ground and has creeping stems with broad leathery leaves that are glossy green on the top and pale and silvery on the underside. Wintergreen has small white flowers followed by edible red berries. The active properties of wintergreen are housed in its leaves.

HISTORICAL NOTES

Native Americans brewed wintergreen leaves into a flavorful and refreshing tea. In colonial times, the leaves were sometimes pounded into a pulp, applied to aching joints, and overwrapped to hold in the heat. This traditional treatment included sipping a cup of wintergreen tea while the poultice did its work. The delicious and flavorful oil distilled from its leaves is very popular— Life Savers and chewing gum come to mind. You might be surprised to know that the volatile oil is also used in some perfumes.

Wintergreen berries, which are sweet, tender, full of flavor— and totally nonmedicinal—were once sold as a natural confection at farmer's markets throughout New England.

SCIENTIFIC FINDINGS

Wintergreen contains methyl salicylate, a relative of aspirin.

TRADITIONAL USE

Internal. To brew wintergreen tea, pour 4 ounces of freshly boiled water over 1/2 teaspoon (1/12 ounce or 2 grams) of the dried leaves. Cover, steep for 3 minutes, and strain. (For more information on brewing teas, see Chapter 3.) Remember, wintergreen is a bitter herb. Add a teaspoon of honey, if you like. Take sparingly.

External. For a warming, pain-relieving treatment for aching muscles or painful, swollen joints, try a pulped poultice of the crushed leaves. You'll find directions for preparing poultices in Chapter 3.

CONSIDERATIONS

Wintergreen is considered a potent herb with the ability to exert a penetrating effect on every cell in the body. It's best to take this herb in the traditional wineglassful doses, a scant half cup.

Yerba mate *(Ilex paraguayensis)*

Yerba mate, pronounced herba-mah-tay, is a traditional herbal brew taken throughout the South American countries. In some areas, it is the national drink, more popular than coffee or any other type of tea.

This herb is a powerful stimulant with tonic, diuretic, and diaphoretic action. It is said to cleanse the blood, tone the nervous system, stimulate the mind, fight fatigue, and ease stress. Yerba mate is even credited with age-retarding properties. It is prescribed to treat arthritis, headache, constipation, and allergies. As an aid to weight-loss, its historic ability to control appetite and its diuretic properties are considered valuable.

Yerba mate tea is said to be very sustaining. On long journeys, country people may carry this herb, taking no refreshment other than the tea for several days with no apparent ill effects.

DESCRIPTION AND PARTS USED

There are many members of the *Ilex* family, including the familiar Christmas holly. *Ilex paraguayensis* grows wild near streams and rivers, although these days it is widely cultivated. It is a handsome shrub that puts forth large white flowers, but it is grown for its leaves. The leaves alternate on the stem and are large, oval, and broadly toothed. Harvested from December to August, the leaves are heat-dried and powdered. Paraguay annually exports millions of pounds of *cha mate* (mate tea) to its South American neighbors.

HISTORICAL NOTES

The name *Yerba* signifies this is an herb of excellence. *Mate* refers to the vessel in which this herb was once brewed. In the ancient manner, the brewed tea was sipped through a straw of silver that was fitted with a strainer on the end. The brewing vessel was passed round the table in a friendly manner and everyone took a pull on the same silver tube. Like many teas, this brew is traditionally flavored with lemon or sugar, except the sugar is caramelized or burnt before being added.

SCIENTIFIC FINDINGS

When fresh yerba mate leaves were dried at Cambridge University in England a while back, the researchers identified caffeine, tannin, ash, and insoluble matter. Other constituents that have since been identified include chlorophyll, iron, trace minerals, and the vitamins B5, C, and E.

TRADITIONAL USE

Internal. If you want to enjoy yerba mate as our South American cousins do, take the tea they call cha mate instead of the beverage you usually consume throughout the day. To make the tea, brew 2 to 3 tablespoons (4/5 to 1 1/5 ounces or 24 to 36 grams) of yerba mate in 16 ounces of freshly boiled water. (For more information on brewing teas, see Chapter 3.) Some find the odor of this herb objectionable and the taste is undeniably bitter, but the stimulating jolt cha mate delivers in each cup is remarkable. Try a cup, flavored with lemon or burnt sugar in the traditional manner, and arrive at your own conclusions.

CONSIDERATIONS

None of the sources I consulted listed any adverse effects from yerba mate. However, it is a powerful stimulant. Sip slowly and monitor your personal reactions.

7

Conclusion

The benefits of twentieth century medicine are many and varied. There's a lot more to applaud than to decry. For example, we have seen stunning advances in orthodox medicine, including monumental technological achievements, near-miraculous surgical techniques, vaccines that protect against what used to be the killer diseases of childhood, and the development of a host of wonder-drugs. As you know, many of our modern drugs originated in the plant kingdom. Not so very long ago, the botanist, pharmacist, and physician were one and the same. As time ticked by, the botanist was bypassed and pharmaceutical companies took over. Busy physicians now often rely on pharmaceutical company's sales representatives to tell them what works.

THE BALANCING ACT

Although none of us wants to return to a time when the only available medicines came from the garden, it's common knowledge that far too many of today's drugs are so harsh, so powerful, that they have toxic side effects. It's been said that adverse drug reactions are becoming so common that almost every patient will experience one sooner or later. That's why treating with manmade pharmaceuticals has become a balancing act. The hope is that the patient can tolerate some of the awful side effects of a more potent drug long enough for it to work and then stop taking the medication before it does irreparable harm.

In today's world, there's a place for knowledgeable and educated physicians with their arsenal of drugs, technological marvels, and advanced surgical techniques just as there is a place for knowledgeable and educated self-care health-care. In my family, we try to combine the best of both. That's a balancing act, too.

I certainly don't want to have a broken bone set on a kitchen table by lantern light, even if comfrey—which Native Americans once called "knit bone"—is simmering on the hob preparatory to making a poultice. If I break a bone, I want it set in a nice clean hospital, and I want a nice clean cast applied until the bone knits straight and true. I don't want to home-treat anything as serious as pneumonia either. I want that potent super-drug and I want oxygen at my hospital bedside, in case it's needed.

Still, I recognize that the human body is a marvelous piece of engineering. We have a lot of finely-tuned self-regulating internal mechanisms designed to protect us. When anything goes wrong, the defensive forces of the body mobilize immediately to deal with the problem. Even before you know something has gone awry, your body is working to correct it. But it's your responsibility to support your body in ways that facilitate healing.

For example, when someone in our family has a sinus infection, we support the body with gentle alternative measures, including healing teas, a salt-solution spritz up the nostrils, hot compresses, and a light diet free of dairy products. We try to avoid the overuse of antibiotics, which, incidentally are not as effective as they once were. You probably already know there's a whole new generation of "bugs" out there that have learned how to beat the drugs that once destroyed them easily (see inset on page 222).

Prevention always will be worth a pound of cure. Ideally, you have adopted a thoughtful lifestyle that promotes a healthy body and wards off problems. You know how important a nutritionally complete diet, coupled with regular and moderate exercise, can be to maintaining your health and extending your life span to the fullest. There's no lack of information on how to accomplish these things so I won't belabor the point here.

When you decide to take a more active role in your own health care, it is your responsibility to know about the effects of the remedies you choose so that you can use them carefully and effectively. I don't believe I have to tell you that it would be foolish in the extreme to self-diagnose and self-treat a serious disease with healing teas alone.

Be aware, also, that just because something is "natural," it doesn't automatically follow that the substance is completely safe. When used appropriately, herbs have a remarkably good record, but not all plants are inoffensive. Data from poison centers nationwide indicates that plants caused one death in 1988 and one in 1989, the last years for which figures are available. There is no indication—*none*—that these deaths were due to any medicinal herbs. In the same two years, poison centers received calls about only two herbs: capsicum and schefflera, which are both considered nontoxic. The problem caused by capsicum was related to juice in a person's eyes. If you can imagine getting jalapeno pepper juice in your eyes, you can well understand the nature of the problem. The plant responsible for the most calls by far to poison centers was the philodendron, with a record of 12,613 accidental poisonings in a single year. Diffenbachia came in second that year with 7,855 reports of poisonings.

Still, you must remember that herbs are powerful pharmaceuticals in their own right. I have carefully selected the natural medicinals included in this book for the brewing of healing teas. In all instances, I have given you the best information available for suggested usage. Some teas have not been included here because they are more toxic than others. Other brews may be toxic if taken in excess, and some of the natural medicinals should only be taken on the advice of a competent health professional well versed in herbology.

Here's something else to remember: Mother Nature isn't required to follow a rule book. There are differences among plants, even those that grow side by side. This means the dried herb you purchase from one source will have a different potency and exhibit different properties from the dried herb you purchase elsewhere. There's no way to standardize the properties of plant pharmaceuticals.

I have only been able to barely touch on the many complexities of the 5,000-year-old healing systems that form the foundation of the healing teas. In truth, as you have seen, many medicinal brews are as effective today as they were centuries ago. For further

Antibiotics Lose Some "Anti"

Perhaps you're not aware that there's a huge problem looming just over the horizon that is threatening our perception of health-care. Some of the so-called wonder-drugs aren't working as well as they once did. Some aren't working at all. The "bugs" are getting smarter. Simply put, many bacteria have learned how to defend themselves against the various drugs that once destroyed them so easily. They have evolved into new and different strains that the drugs can't touch. This sorry state of affairs came about because of the over-use of antibiotics.

We can't put all the blame on the scientists and the medical profession either. First, no one dreamed the "bugs" would outsmart the drugs. Second, a lot of it is our fault. See if these little scenarios ring true:

"I have a really awful sore throat, doctor, but I can't afford to take time off work. Can't you just give me an antibiotic?"

"That same tooth is acting up again, doc, and it really hurts. Can I have some of the antibiotic that cleared up the infection before?"

"My child has another earache, doctor; would you please call in a prescription for the antibiotic that worked last time?"

"I know my sinuses are infected, doctor. Can I just come in and pick up a prescription for an antibiotic?"

If any of these statements sound even vaguely familiar, you'll realize that we have come to rely heavily on the wonder-drugs.

Unfortunately, overexposure to antibiotics is commonplace. Because they have entered the food chain, we can't always avoid antibiotics, even when we make the effort. Dairy cows and meat animals, including poultry, are routinely injected with antibiotics or given the drugs in their feed to keep them healthy and ready for market. As a result, milk, meat, and poultry all carry traces of the drugs. If you are drinking milk or eating meat or poultry, you're "taking" antibiotics. I'm a big believer in preventive health-care. However, in this case, that dose of preventive medicine given to animals can end up working against us.

Those in the know try to steer clear of antibiotics and reserve their use for something serious, like pneumonia, for example. We're trying to stay ahead of the game in case a serious condition does arise that warrants the use of an antibiotic. Is this a reasonable premise? I'm not sure.

Should a family member come down with something serious, we'll just have to hope, first, that the bacteria causing the disease hasn't evolved into one of the nasty drug-resistant strains, and, second, that the drug will work because that person has not been overexposed to antibiotics.

insight, read up on the subject. Browse through the books on natural healing in your library or local book shop. Take home one or two, curl up on the sofa with a cup of tea, open the book, and enjoy!

To experience the intricacies of an herbal formula precisely tailored to your body, you might consult a master herbalist the next time you have a problem. What's that? You don't have an herbalist in your rolodex? No problem. In most cities, you'll find herbalists listed in the yellow pages of your local telephone book under "Herbs." I suggest you introduce yourself to the herbalist by phone and select the one who seems most sympathetic and knowledgeable. In the hands of a true master herbalist, you will have a fascinating consultation and careful exploration of your problem. Most of the time, you'll come home with a blend of natural medicinals that will brew into a marvelously healing tea.

Because there's no way to adequately explain how the various herbs interact with one another, or predict how they might react with your personal body chemistry, I have not included combination formulas. I favor the simple approach of brewing one-ingredient teas. If this book does nothing more than encourage you to take a pleasant cup of healing tea the next time you're under the weather, I will be pleased.

In the foregoing pages, you've seen how the millennia-old art of brewing healing teas can be relevant in your life today. Although it is not the case in this country, worldwide, more people use natural medicinals—primarily in the form of herbal brews—than rely on prescription drugs. We may be approaching a time when it makes sense to take advantage of some of the simple remedies of yesterday.

I hope you have enjoyed this amble through the history of healing teas as much as I have enjoyed bringing it to you. There are many excellent books that cover the ancient alternative therapies, including the brewing of healing teas. Each one is more fascinating than the last. Delve deep.

Sources
of Supplies

Sipping teas can be found in almost any supermarket or health-food store. For loose medicinal herbs, herbal tea combination formulas, and/or medicinal herbs in teabags, or for information on the preceding, contact:

Crystal Star Herbal Nutrition
14409 Cuesta Court
Sonora, California 95370
(209) 532-6474

Frontier Cooperative Herbs
3021 78th Street
P.O. Box 118
Norway, Iowa 52318-0118
(800) 786-1388

San Francisco Herb Co.
250 14th Street
San Francisco, CA 94103
(800) 227-4530
(415) 861-7174

Seelect Herb Tea Company
P.O. Box 1969
Camarillo, CA 93011
(805) 484-0899

For a free information packet or to purchase a kombucha mushroom starter kit, contact:

Laurel Farms
P.O. Box 7405
Studio City, CA 91614
(213) 650-1060

For a complete list of preblended healing teas, plus other product information, and a list of local shops carrying Traditional Medicinal teas, contact:

Natural Resources
6680 Harvard Drive
Sebastopol, CA 95472
(800) 747-0390

For the legendary teas of India, China, Ceylon, Africa, Taiwan, and Japan, as well as fruited and spiced teas, teapots, tea sets (including miniatures), tea cozies, and more, contact:

Windham Tea Company
12 Wilson Road
Windham, NH 03087
(800) 565-7527

Sources
of Information

Burgeoning interest in alternative healing methods os reflected by the wealth of information available.

SCIENTIFIC DATA

For solid scientific material on the natural healing herbs, contact:

The Herb Research Foundation
1007 Pearl Street
Suite 200
Boulder, Colorado 80302
(303) 449-2265
www.herbs.org

HERBAL TEAS

To quickly find shops or mail order sources for seeds, plants, brewing herbs, and much, much more, I recommend:

The Herb Companion Wish Book & Resource Guide by Bobbi A. McRae.
To order, contact:

Interweave Press
201 E. Fourth Street
Loveland, CO 80537
(800) 272-2193

INDIAN HEALING TEAS

For information on the Ayuvedic healing teas of India and other herbal product, or for a free mind-body dosha evaluation, contact:

Maharashi Ayur-Ved Products, Inc.
P.O. Box 49667

Colorado Springs, CO 80949-9667
(800) 255-8332

For information on Ayurvedic teas, yogi teas, herbal formulas, even massage oils, contact:

Ancient Healing Ways
Route 3, Box 259
Espanola, New Mexico 87532
(800) 359-2940

For mail-order service, beautifully illustrated literature, and solid information on the legendary Chinese tonic teas plus books on the healing teas of many cultures, contact:

The Tea Garden Herbal Emporium
Suite 200
903 Colorado Avenue
Santa Monica, CA 90401
(310) 205-0104

CANADIAN HEALING TEAS

For fully-researched information on Rene Caisse's cancer formula, I recommend:

Options: The Alternative Cancer Therapy Book by Richard Walters.

To order, contact:

Avery Publishing Group
120 Old Broadway
Garden City Park, NY 11040
(800) 548-5757

For information on essiac and other Canadian healing teas, contact:

Ontario Herbalists' Association
11 Winthrop Place
Stoney Creek, Ontario
L8G 3M3 Canada
(416) 536-1509

MACROBIOTICS

For referral to a counselor or teacher in your area who is fully trained in the macrobiotic way, contact:

The Kushi Institute
Box 7
Lealand Road
Becket, MA 01223
(413) 623-5742

Vega Study Center
1511 Robinson Street
Oroville, CA 95965
(916) 533-4777

Bibliography

Abravanel, Elliot D. *Dr. Abravanel's Body Type Program for Health, Fitness and Nutrition*. New York: Bantam Books, 1986.

Adams, Ruth. "Healthful Herb Teas." *Better Nutrition for Today's Living*, July 1993, 40–44.

——. "The Healing Power of Herb Teas," *Better Nutrition for Today's Living*, June 1992, 31–33.

Airola, Paavo. *Worldwide Secrets for Staying Young*. Phoenix, Arizona: Health Plus Publishers, 1982.

Balch, James F. and Phyllis A. Balch. *Prescription for Nutritional Healing*. Garden City Park, New York: Avery Publishing, 1990.

Begley, Sharon. *"Beyond Vitamins,"* *Newsweek*, April 25, 1994, 45–49.

Bricklin, Mark, ed. *The Practical Encyclopedia of Natural Healing*. Emmaus, Pennsylvania: Rodale Press, Inc., 1976.

Budwig, Johanna. *Flax Oil as a True Aid Against Arthritis, Heart Infarction, Cancer, and Other Diseases*. Vancouver, British Columbia: Apple Publishing Co., 1992.

Carper, Jean. *The Food Pharmacy*. New York: Bantam Books, 1989.

Chopra, Deepak. *Quantum Healing*. New York: Bantam Books, 1989.

Clark, Linda. *Get Well Naturally*. New York, Arco Publishing Co., Inc., 1974.

Columbia-Viking Desk Encyclopedia. New York: Viking Press, 1960.

Coon, Nelson. *Using Plants for Healing*. Emmaus, Pennsylvania: Rodale Press, 1979.

Davis, Adelle. *Let's Get Well*. Chicago, Illinois: Signet Books, 1972.

Duke, James A., ed. *CRC Handbook of Medicinal Herbs*. Boca Raton, Florida: CRC Press, Inc., 1985.

Family Guide to Natural Medicine: How to Stay Healthy the Natural Way. Pleasantville, New York: Reader's Digest Association, 1993.

Foster, Steven. *Milk Thistle: Silybum marianum*. Austin, Texas: American Botanical Council, Series No. 305.

Frazier, Cynthia. "It Comes Naturally." *The Outlook* (Santa Monica, CA), March 27, 1994, B1.

Glanze, Walter D., ed. *Signet/Mosby Medical Encyclopedia*. New York: Signet Books, 1987.

Grieve, Mrs. M. *A Modern Herbal*. New York: Dover Publications, 1971.

Hsu, Hong-Yen. *Chinese Herb Medicine & Therapy*. Hawaiian Gardens, California: Oriental Healing Arts Institute of U.S.A., 1976.

Hylton, William H. *Rodale Herb Book*. Emmaus, Pennsylvania: Rodale Press Book Division, 1974.

Jizong, Shi and Chu Feng Zhu. *The ABC of Traditional Chinese Medicine*. Hong Kong: Hai Feng Publishing Company, 1985.

Kloss, Jethro. *Back to Eden*. Loma Linda, California: Eden Books, 1985.

Kowalchik, Claire and William H. Hylton, eds. *Rodale's Illustrated*

Encyclopedia of Herbs. Emmaus, Pennsylvania: Rodale Press, 1987.

Kushi, Micho. *How to See Your Health: Book of Oriental Diagnosis.* Tokyo: Japan Publications, Inc., 1980.

——. *The Macrobiotic Way.* Garden City Park, New York: Avery Publishing Group, 1993.

Lathrop, Norma Jean. *Herbs: How to Select, Grow and Enjoy.* Tucson, Arizona: H.P. Books, 1981.

Lessel, Colin B. *Homeopathy for Physicians.* Wellingborough, Northamptonshire, England: Thorsons Publishers Ltd., 1983.

Levy, Juliette de Bairacli. *Herbal Handbook for Farm and Stable.* Great Britain: Faber and Faber, Ltd., 1952

Lu, Henry C. *Chinese System of Food Cures, Prevention & Remedies,* New York: Sterling Publishing Co., Inc., 1986.

Lucas, Richard Melvin. *Herbal Health Secrets From Europe and Around the World,* New York: Parker Publishing Co., Inc., 1983.

Magic Herbs for Arthritis, Rheumatism, and Related Ailments. New York: Parker Publishing Co., Inc., 1981.

Magic of Herbs in Daily Living, The. New York: Parker Publishing Co., Inc., 1972.

McCaleb, Robert S. *Herb Safety Report.* Herb Research Foundation: Boulder, Colorado, 1993.

McRae, Bobbi A. *The Herb Companion, Wishbook and Resource Guide.* Loveland, Colorado: Interweave Press, 1992.

Mindell, Earl. *Earl Mindell's Herb Bible.* New York: Simon & Schuster, 1992.

Murray, Frank. "The Best of Herb Teas." *Better Nutrition for Today's Living* 55 (February 1993): 46–49.

Murray, Michael T. *The Healing Power of Herbs.* Rocklin, California: Prima Publishing, 1992.

Nutrition Almanac. 2d ed. New York: McGraw-Hill, 1984.

Pahlow, Mannfried. *Living Medicine: The Healing Properties of*

Plants. Wellingborough, Northamptonshire, England: Thorsons Publishers Limited, 1980.

Pearson, Durk and Sandy Shaw. *Life Extension: A Practical Scientific Approach*. New York: Warner Books, 1982.

Pedersen, Mark. *Nutritional Herbology*. Bountiful, Utah: Pedersen Publishing, 1987.

Physicians' Desk Reference. 35th ed. Oradell, New Jersey: Medical Economics Data, 1981.

Pizzorno, Jr., Joseph E., N.D., and Michael T. Murray, N.D. *A Textbook of Natural Medicine*. Seattle, Washington: John Bastyr College Publications, 1985.

Revolutionary Health Committee of Hunan Province, The. *A Barefoot Doctor's Manual*. Seattle, Washington: Madrona Publishers, 1977.

Santillo, Humbart. *Herbal Combinations from Authoritative Sources*. 3rd ed. Provo, Utah: NuLife Publishing, Inc., 1983.

Schultes, Richard Evans and Albert Hofmann. *Plants of the Gods*. Maidenhead, England: McGraw-Hill Book Company (UK) Limited, 1979.

Sharma, Hari, M.D. *Freedom From Disease*. Toronto: Veda Publishing, 1993.

Snow, Shiela. "Old Ontario Remedies: Essiac." *Canadian Journal of Herbalism*, 1991, 1–3.

Steinman, David. "Why You Should Drink Green Tea." *Natural Health*, March/April 1994, 56–58.

Tenney, Louise. *Today's Herbal Health*. 2d ed. Provo, Utah: Woodland Books, 1983.

Thomas, Clayton L., M.D., M.P.H. *Taber's Cyclopedic Medical Dictionary* 12th ed. Philadelphia, Pennsylvania: F.A. Davis Company, 1974.

Tierra, Michael. *The Way of Herbs*. Santa Cruz, California: Unity Press, 1980.

Wade, Carlson. *The Pocket Encyclopedia of Natural Folk Remedies.* New York: Globe Communications, 1979.

Walford, Roy L. *Maximum Life Span.* New York: W. W. Norton & Co., Inc., 1983.

Walters, Richard. *Options: The Alternative Cancer Therapy Book.* Garden City Park, New York: Avery Publishing Group, 1993.

Weil, Andrew. *Health and Healing.* Boston, Massachusetts: Houghton Mifflin Company, 1983.

Willard, Terry, Ph.D. *The Wild Rose Scientific Herbal.* Alberta, Canada: Wild Rose College of Natural Healing, Ltd., 1991.

Zebrowski, Shirley. "Herbal Teas." *Total Health* 15 (February 1993), 36–38.

Index

Abortifacients, 73
Abor-vitae, 73
Acetylsalicylic acid. *See* Aspirin.
Acne, 92
Acupuncture points, 29
Adaptogen, 144
Adrenal-function-related problems, 92
Adrenaline. *See* Epinephrine.
Age-related disorders, 92
AIDS, 92, 208
Alcoholism, 92
Alfalfa, 97–98
Allergies, 92
Allium sativum. *See* Garlic.
Alterative, 73–74
Althea officinalis. See Marshmallow.
American Cancer Society, 45, 151
American colonies, 18–19

Ancient Healing Ways products, 72
Anemia, 92
Angelica, 4, 98–101
Angelica atropurpurea. See Angelica.
Angelica sinensis. See Dong quai.
Anise, 101–103
Anodyne, 74
Anthelmintic, 74
Anthemis nobilis. See Chamomile.
Antibiotics, 222–223
Antipyretic, 74
Antiscorbutic, 74
Antiseptic, 32, 40
Apierient. *See* Laxative.
Arctium lappa. See Burdock.
Arctostaphylos uva ursi. See Uva ursi.
Ardutin, 210

Aristotle, 35
Aromatherapy, 74, 204
Aromatic, 74
Art alcove, Japanese, 15
Arthritis, 92
Asarum canadense. See Ginger,
    wild.
Aspirin, 44, 214
Assam, 10, 17
    tea, 10, 21
    tree, 10
Asthma, 32, 92
Astragalus, 103–104
Astragalus membranaceous.
    See Astragalus.
Astringent, 74
Ayur-Ved. *See* Medicine,
    Indian.

Bakers, Norman, 159
Balm of Giliad, 106
Bancha tea, 43
Barton, Dr., 198
Bath, herbal, 55
Bed-wetting, 92
Bee pollen, 104–107
    candy, 105
Benign prostatic hypertrophy
    (BPH), 199–200
Bererine, 147
Bergamot tree, 12
Bible, 36
    Gutenberg, 38
Black cohosh, 107–109
Black Death. *See* Bubonic
    plague.
Black tea, 11, 12–13, 24, 150
Blechynden, Richard, 19
Blood-pressure-related
    problems, 92

Blood purifiers, 75, 92
Bodhidharma, 15
Boer War, 182
Bone-related problems, 92
Boston Tea Party, 18
BPH. *See* Benign prostatic
    hypertrophy.
Brahmi. *See* Gotu kola.
Breathe Easy tea, 70
British Medical Journal, 119
Bronchitis, 92
Brown, Royden, 105
Bubonic plague, 38
Buckthorn bark, 113
Bugbane. *See* Black cohosh.
Burdock, 109–110, 130
Burkitt, R. W., 131
Burns, 92

Caffeic acid phenethyl ester,
    182
Caisse, Rene, 129
Calendar of the Hsai, 136
Calendula, 110–112
Calendula officinalis. See
    Calendula.
Cambodia, 10
    tree, 10–11
Cambridge University, 218
Camellia sinensis. See Black tea;
    Green tea; Oolong tea.
Camellia sinensis tea plant,
    10
Camphor, 32
Canadian Journal of Herbalism,
    The, 131
Cancer, 92
Candied Sage Leaves, 193
CAPE. *See* Caffeic acid
    phenethyl ester.

Capsicum, 221. *See also*
Cayenne.
Capsicum anuum. See Cayenne.
Capsicum frutescens. See
Cayenne.
Caraway, 74
tea, 36
Carbenoxolone, 163
Carminative, 75
Cascara sagrada, 112–114
Castor oil, 32
Catechins, 50
Cathartic. *See* Laxative.
Catherine of Portugal, 16
Cayenne, 114–115
Centella asiatica. See Gotu kola.
Ceylon Breakfast tea, 21
Ceylon tea, 12, 21
*Chado, The Japanese Way of
Tea* (Soshitsu Sen), 15
Cha-no-yu. *See* Tea, ceremony,
Japanese.
Cha-shitsu. *See* Tearoom,
Japanese.
Chamomile, 4, 20, 49, 116–117
tea, 77
Charaka Samhita, 34
Charlemagne, 170
Charles II (England), 16
Chaulmoogra oil, 32
Chesima tea plant, 11
Chi, 29
China, 10
China Rose tea, 21
Chinese rhubarb, 32
Cholesterol
HDL, 75
LDL, 50
Cholesterol-related problems,
92

Chrysanthemum parthenium. See
Feverfew.
Cimicifuga racemosa. See Black
cohosh.
Cinchona bark, 43, 44
Circulatory-system-related
problems, 92
Citrus bergama. See Bergamot
tree.
Classic of Tea, The (Lu Yu), 14
Cloves, 74
Code of Hammurabi, 37
Codeine, 44
Cold Care P.M. tea, 70
Cold extremities, 92
Colds and flu, 93
Colic, 93
Colon toxicity, 93
Columbia University, 182
Columbus, Christopher, 38
Comfrey, 118–120
Commiphora opobalsamum. See
Balm of Giliad.
Compleat Herbal, A (Culpeper),
39
Congestion, 93
Constipation, 32, 36, 93
Copper, 36
Cordial, 75
Corroborant. *See* Tonic.
Cotton, 73
Coughs, 93
Crescentius, Peter, 38
Crystal Star Herbal Nutrition,
71, 225
Culpeper, Nicholas, 38, 39,
99, 109, 117, 119, 134, 154,
155, 156, 170, 191, 204

Damiana, 120–121

Dandelion, 122–123
  root tea, 43, 74
Dandruff, 93
De Agricultura (Crescentius),
  38
Decoction, 55–56
Deforestation, 45
Deglycyrrhizinated licorice
  (DGL), 163
Demulcent, 75
Dental-related problems, 93
Deobstruent, 75
Depression, 93
Depurant, 75
DGL. *See* Deglycyrrhizinated
  licorice.
DHT. *See* Dihydrotestosterone.
Diabetes, 93
Diaphoretic, 75
Diarrhea, 32, 44, 93
Diffenbachia, 221
Digestion-related problems,
  93
Digitalis, 32
Digitalis purpurea. See Fox-
  glove.
Digitoxin, 43
Dihydrotestosterone (DHT),
  200
Dioscorides, Pedanius, 36,
  117, 214
Distillation, 37
Diuretic, 75
Doctrine of Signatures, 32
Doctrine of the Pulse, 30, 34
Dong quai, 123–124
Dosha, 34
Dramamine, 140
Drugs. *See* Medicines,
  synthetic.

Ear-related problems, 93
Earl Grey Imperial tea. *See*
  Earl Grey tea.
Earl Grey tea, 12, 21
East India Company, 16
East-West Foundation, 43
East-West Journal (East-West
  Foundation), 43
Eccletics, 144
Echinacea, 4, 125–126
Echinacea angustifolia. See
  Echinacea.
Echinacea Fitness Tea, 72
EGCB. *See* Epigallocatechin
  gallate.
Eleutherococcus senticosus. See
  Ginseng, Siberian.
Elizabeth I (England), 16
Emerson, G. B., 197
Emetic, 76
Emmenagogue, 76
Emollient, 76
Endotoxins, 196
English Breakfast tea, 12, 21
English Physician, The
  (Culpeper), 39
Englishman's Doctor, The
  (Harrington), 136
Enquiry Into Plants, An
  (Theophratus), 35
Ephedra, 4, 32. *See also*
  Mahuang.
Ephedra sinica. See Ephedra.
Ephedrine, 32, 168, 169
Epigallocatechin gallate
  (EGCG), 151
Epilepsy, 93
Epinephrine, 168
Equisetum arvense. See
  Horsetail.

Essiac, 129–133
Euphrasia officinalis. See
   Eyebright.
Expectorant, 76
Eyebright, 127–128
Eye-related problems, 93

Farbenfabriken Bayer
   Aktiengegesellschaft, 214
Fatigue
   mental, 93
   physical, 93
FDA. *See* U.S. Food and Drug
   Administration.
Febrifuge, 76
Female disorders, 93
Fever, 93
Feverfew, 133–135
   tea, 3, 4
Flatulence. *See* Gas.
Fletcher's Castoria, 113
Flu. *See* Colds and flu.
Fomentation, 57
Food and Drug Adminis-
   tration, U.S., 70, 107
Foxglove, 32, 43
Frangelica, 100
Frankincense, 37
Fu Hsi, 31
Fungus Japonicus. See Kom-
   bucha.

Galen, 35, 214
Gallbladder-related problems,
   94
Gallstones, 94
Garden of Pleasure (Parkinson),
   203
Garlic, 136–139
   syrup, 138

Gas, 94
Gastrointestinal problems, 94
Gaultheria procumbens. See
   Wintergreen.
Gerald's Herbal, 38, 102
Gerard, John, 97, 133, 154,
   176, 191, 203
Ginger, 139–141
   root, 4, 74
   wild, 140
Ginkgo, 141–142
   biloa extract, 142
Ginkgo biloba. See Ginkgo.
Ginseng, 4, 32
   American, 143–145
   Chinese, 143–145
   Energy, 72
   Korean, 143–145
   Siberian, 143–145
"Ginseng Abuse Syndrome"
   (JAMA), 145
Glum, Gary L., Dr., 131
Glutathione, 172
Glycyrrhetic acid, 163
Glycyrrhiza glabra. See Licorice.
Glycyrrhizin, 163, 164
Golden Green Tea, 70
Goldenseal, 4, 32, 146–148
Gotu kola, 148–150
Gout, 94
Great Pharmacopoeia (Li
   Shih-chen), 31
Green tea, 11, 24, 70,
   150–153, 168
Guaiac, 38
Gutenberg, Johann, 38

Hair-related problems, 94
Harrington, John, Sir, 136
Headache, 94

migraine, 94
Healing teas, 27
  Ancient tradition of, 27–28,
    29–37
  function of, 51–52
  in colonial America, 40–42
  macrobiotic way and,
    42–43
  medicine and, 28–29, 37–40,
    43–44
  modern use of, 44–45,
    47–66
  preparing, 52–66
  shopping for, 67–78
  terminology, 73–78
Health and Healing (Weil), 48
Heart problems, 94
Heartburn, 94
Hemorrhoids, 94
Henbane, 36
Hepatic, 76
*The Herb Companion: Wishbook
  and Resource Guide*
  (McRae), 69, 227
Herb cultivation, 79
  drying, 85–86
  growing medium, 82–83
  harvesting, 84–85
  planters for, 79–81
  selecting plants for, 83–84
  storing dried herbs, 86–87
Herb teas, 20–21, 24, 25. *See
  also* Teas, healing.
Herbs, whole
  measuring, 53–54
  preparing, 52–66
  shopping for, 67–78
  synthetic medicines and,
    47–50, 219–224
High blood pressure, 32, 94

High tea, 17–18
Hippocrates, 42, 102, 106, 214
HIV, 208
Holy wood. *See* Guaiac.
Horehound, 153–156
  cough and cold syrup, 155
Horsetail, 156–157
Hot flashes, 187
Huang-di, 31
Huang Ti, 31
Hufeland, Christophe W., 42
Human immunodeficiency
  virus. *See* HIV.
Hydrastis canadensis. See
  Goldenseal.
Hydroquinone, 210, 211
Hyoscyamus. *See* Henbane.
Hypericum perforatum. See St.
  John's wort.
Hypoglycemia, 2, 94

Iced tea, 19
  Thai, 26
Ilex paraguayensis. See Yerba
  mate.
Immune-function-related
  problems, 94
Indian tea, 12
Indigestion, 36
Industrial Revolution, 186
Infection, 94
Infusion, 57
  cold, 57
  hot and cold, 58–59
Insect bites and stings, 94
Insomnia, 49, 94
Ipe Roxo. *See* Pau d'Arco.
Ipecac, 36
Irish Breakfast tea, 12, 21
Iron, 32

JAMA. *See* Journal of the American *Medical Association.*
Jasmine tea, 21
John the Baptist, 206
Josselyn, John, 40
Journal of Bioscience, 115
Journal of Medical Chemistry, 126
Journal of New Chinese Medicine, 140
Journal of the American Medical Association, 145
Journal of the Japanese Society of Food Science and Technology, 152
Juice, herbal, 60
Juniper, 73

Kaolin, 32
Kapha dosha, 34
Kapha tea, 72
Kargasok tea. *See* Kombucha tea.
Keemun tea, 21
Keratin, 32
Kidney-related problems, 94
Kombu, Dr., 160
Kombu tea, 43
Kombucha, 158–161
tea, 159–160
Kushi, Michio, 43
Kushi Institute, 43

L-dopa, 209
Lancet, 131, 134, 135
LaPacho. *See* Pau d'Arco.
Lapsang Souchong tea, 21
Laudanum, 44
Laxative, 76
Lemon tea, 21, 74

Leprosy, 32
Leroux, 214
Lethargy, 94
Leung, Albert, Dr., 140
LiChing Yun, 149
Li Shih-chen, 31
Lice, 94
Licorice, 4, 162–164
Lipton, Thomas, 13
Lipton Tea Company, 13
Lister, Joseph, Baron, 40
Liver-related problems, 95
Lobelia, 164–165, 167
plant, 32
Lobelia inflata. See Lobelia.
Lobeline, 165
London Migraine Clinic, 135
London Pharmacopoeia, 39, 210
Louis XIV (France), 16
Low blood pressure, 95
Low Blood Sugar and You, 2
Lu Yu, 14
Lung-related problems, 95
Lythontryptic, 76

McRae, Bobbi A., 69
Macrobiotics, 42–43
Macrobiotics, or The Art of Prolonging Life (Hufeland), 42
Maharishi Ayur-Ved Teas, 72
Mahuang, 167–169 *See also* Ephedra.
Male disorders, 95
Male Vitality Tea, 72
Maleria, 43, 44
Mallow, 75
Malva. See Mallow.
Manchurian tea. *See* Kombucha tea.

Marigold. *See* Calendula.
Marrubium vulgare. See Horehound.
Marshmallow, 75, 169–171
Mary's sweat, 208
Materia Medica (Dioscorides), 36
Materia Medica (Gerard), 203
Mather, Cotton, 134, 135
Matricaria chamomilla. See Chamomile.
Medicago sativa. See Alfalfa.
Medicine
    allopathic, 50
    American colonial, 40–42
    Arabian, 37
    changing face of, 39–40
    Chinese, 29–31
    Egyptian, 36
    European, 37–39
    Greek, 35–36
    herbal teas as, 43–44
    Indian, 33–35
    Roman, 35–36
    Western, 28–29
Medicines, synthetic, compared with natural medicinals, 47–50, 219–224
Mentha piperita. See Peppermint.
Mentha spicata. See Spearmint.
Meridians, 29
Metamucil, 183
Methyl salicylate, 216
Migraine. *See* Headache, migraine.
Milk thistle, 171–173
Mint, 74

Mitchella repens. See Squawvine.
Mo Ching, 31
Monardes, Nicholas, 38
Monks
    Buddhist, 14
    Zen, 15
Morning sickness, 188
Morphine, 44
Motion sickness, 95
Mu tea, 43
Mullein, 173
Muscle cramps, 95
Mushroom of long life. *See* Kombucha tea.
Myrrh, 37

Nail-related problems, 95
National Cancer Institute, 45
National Formulary, 215
Nausea, 95
Nei Ching (Huang-di), 31, 32
Nervine, 76–77
Nervous-system-related problems, 95
New England Rarities Discovered... (Josselyn), 41
New York University Medical Center, 208
Night sweats, 95
Nursing-related problems, 95
Nutmeg, 74

Ohsawa, George, 43
Oil, herbal, 60
Ointment, herbal, 61
"Old Ontario Remedies: 1922: Rene Caisse: Essiac" (*The Canadian Journal of Herbalism*), 131

Oolong tea, 11–12, 24
Opium poppy, 44, 74
Options: The Alternative Cancer Therapy Book (Walters), 131
Orange pekoe tea, 12. *See also* Black tea.
Orris root, 204
Ottawa Department of Health and Welfare, 129
The Outlook, 159
Oxytocic. *See* Parturient.

Pacific yew tree, 44
Pain, 95
Palo santo. *See* Guaiac.
Panax ginseng. See Ginseng, Chinese; Ginseng, Korean.
Pancreas-related problems, 95
Panex quinquefolius. See Ginseng, American.
Papaver somniferum. See Opium poppy.
Paregoric, 44
Parkinson, John, 109, 174, 176, 203
Parsley, 175–177
Parturient, 77
Pau d'Arco, 70, 178–179
Pectoral, 77
Pekoe, 12. *See also* Black tea.
Pen-ts-ao Kang-mu. See Great Pharmacopeia.
Pennyroyal, 73
People magazine, 158
Peppermint, 179–181
Petroselinum crispum. See Parsley.
Pharmaceutical Society of Great Britain, 39

Philodendron, 221
Physicians of Myddfai, 210
Pillow, herbal, 204–205
Pimpinella anisum. See Anise.
Pimples. *See* Skin conditions.
Pingsuey tea, 21
Pitta dosha, 34
Pitta Tea, 72
Planta Medica, 126
Plantago psyllium. See Psyllium.
Plaster, herbal, 61
Plato, 35
Pliny the Elder, 36, 106, 117
PMS Tea, 70
Polyphenols, 151
Potentiator, 77
Potter's Cyclopaedia of Botanical Drugs and Preparations, 121, 211–212
Potting soil, super-charged, 83
Poultice
  herbal, pulped, 61–63
  herbal, steamed, 63–65
Prince of Wales tea, 21
Propolis, 4, 181–183
  tea, 4
Pryor, Betsy, 159
Pseudoephedrine, 168
Psyllium, 183–185
Pulse Classic. *See Mo Ching.*
Purgative. *See* Laxative.
Pustules. *See* Skin conditions.

Quinine, 43, 44

Rain Forest Action Coalition, 45
Raphael, Archangel, 99
Rasayana, 34

Amrit Nectar, 35
Rash. *See* Skin conditions.
Rauwolfia, 32
Red clover, 185–186
Red raspberry, 187–188
Resperin Corporation of
    Ontario, 129
Rhamnus catharica. See Buck-
    thorn bark.
Rhamnus purshiana. See
    Cascara sagrada.
Rheum palmatum. See Turkey
    rhubarb.
Rheumatism, 95
Rice tea, 43
Rich Sage Tea, 192
Roasted barley tea, 43
Robinson, William, Dr., 107
Rose hips, 20, 188–190
*Royden Brown's Bee Hive
    Product Bible* (Brown), 105
Rubefacient, 77
Rubus idaeus. See Red rasp-
    berry.
Rumex acetosella. See Sheep's
    sorrel.
Russian Caravan tea, 21
Russian penicillin. *See*
    Propolis.
Russian tea, 21

Safrole, 198
Sage, 190–194
    Leaves, Candied, 193
    tea. *See* Rich Sage Tea.
Sagen Ishizuka, Dr., 42
Salicin, 44, 214
Salicylic acid, 44, 214
Salix. See Willow.
Salix alba. See White willow.

Salve, herbal, 65–66
Salvia officinalis. See Sage.
Sarsaparilla, 38, 74, 194–196
Sassafras, 197–198
    oil, 198
Sassafras officinale. See Sassa-
    fras.
Sauce Saracen, 189
Sauce Sarzyn. *See* Sauce
    Saracen.
Saw palmetto, 198–200
Scales, 53–54
Schefflera, 221
Scopolamine, 36
Scouring brush. *See*
    Horsetail.
Scutellaria lateriflora. See Skull-
    cap.
Sedative, 77
Seelect Herb Tea Company,
    71
Semi-fermented teas, brewing,
    24
Sen Rikyu, 15
Serenoa repens. See Saw
    palmetto.
Sex-related problems, 95
Shaker apothecaries, 41–42
Sheep's sorrel, 130
Shen-Nung, 14, 26, 31
Shennong Herbal, 149, 162
Silybum marianum. See Milk
    thistle.
Silymarin, 171, 172, 173
Sinusitis, 95
Sipping teas, 9
    brewing, 22–24
    composition of, 13–14
    description of, 10–11
    history of, 14–19

processing, 11–13
taste of, 19–20, 21
time for, 25–26
traditional (table), 21
Skin conditions, 95
Sklenar, Rudolph, Dr., 161
Skota. *See* Skunk cabbage.
Skullcap, 201–202
Skunk cabbage, 74
Slippery elm, 130
Smilax officinalis. See Sarsaparilla.
Smithsonian Report, 197
Smoking, problems quitting, 95
Smooth Move Tea, 70
Society of Apothecaries, 39
Sore throat, 96
Spasms, 96
uterine, 187
Spearmint, 202–205
Spikenard. *See* Valerian.
Spoons, 54
perforated, 22
Squawvine, 166
Squill, 36
St. John's wort, 49, 205–209
oil, 207–208
St. Louis Fair (1904), 19
Stimulant, 77
Stinkweed. *See* Garlic.
Stomachic, 77
Stone, Reverend, 214
Strawberry barrel, 80, 81
how to fill, 82
Strawberry pot, 80
Stress, 96
Stroke, 96
Sublimination, 37
Sudorific. *See* Diaphoretic.

Sullivan, Thomas, 19
Susruta Samhita, 149
Sweetflag, 74
Symphytum officinale. See Comfrey.
Syphilis, 38, 195

Tabebuia avellanedae. See Pau d'Arco.
Tansy, 73
Taraxacum officinale. See Dandelion.
Taxol, 44
Tea
bag, 19
ball, 22
ceremony, Japanese, 14
mug, 22
strainer, 23
time, 25–26
traders, 16–17
tradition, Japanese, 14–16
Teapots, 23
Tearoom, Japanese, 15
Thebaine, 44
Theocretus, 176
Theophylline, 168
Thomson, Samuel, 164, 165
Thyme tea, 77
Tics, 96
Tincture, 66, 69
Toko-no-ma. *See* Art alcove, Japanese.
Tonic, 77–78
Torah, 36
Toyotomi Hideyoshi, 15
Traditional Medicinals Herb Tea Company, 70
Trees and Shrubs of Massachusetts (Emerson), 197

Trepanning, 28
Trifolium pratense. See Red
    clover.
Tryptophan, 209
Turkey rhubarb, 130–131
Turnera aphrodisiaca. See
    Damiana.
Tyramine, 209

Ulcers, 96
Ulmus fulva. See Slippery elm.
Umeboshi tea, 43
United States Dispensatory, 214
United States Pharmacopeia,
147, 165, 180, 198, 214
University of California
    (Davis), 50
University of California
    (Los Angeles), 115
University of Texas (Hous-
    ton), 104
Urinary-tract-related prob-
    lems, 96
U.S. Food and Drug Admini-
    stration (FDA), 70, 107
USA Today, 158
Uva ursi, 76, 209–211

Vaidya, 34
Valerian, 4, 49–50, 76–77,
    211–213
Valeriana officinalis. See
    Valerian.
Varicose veins, 96
Vata dosha, 34

Vata tea, 72
Venereal diseases, 96
Verbascum thapsus. See
    Mullein.
Verdigris, 36
Vermifuges, 74
Verodoxin, 32
Vespetro, 100
Vomiting, 96
Vulnerary, 78

Water retention, 96
Waterhouse, Andrew, Dr.,
    50
Weight control, 96
Weil, Andrew, Dr., 48
Weizmann Institute of
    Science (Israel), 208
Whitaker, 40
White willow, 213–215
Willow, 44, 74
Willow bark tea, 73
Winter tonic, 166
Wintergreen, 215–217
Women's Tea, 72
Wounds, 96

Yeast infections, 96
Yerba mate, 217–218
Yin and yang, 29
Yukikazu Sakurazawa, 42
Yunnan tea, 21

Zingiber officinales. See
    Ginger.

Healthy Habits

are easy to come by—

IF YOU KNOW WHERE TO LOOK!

Get the latest information on:

- **better health • diet & weight loss**
- **the latest nutritional supplements**
- **herbal healing • homeopathy and more**

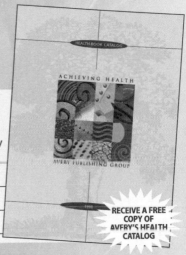

RECEIVE A FREE
COPY OF
AVERY'S HEALTH
CATALOG

COMPLETE AND RETURN THIS CARD RIGHT AWAY!

Where did you purchase this book?

❑ bookstore   ❑ health food store   ❑ pharmacy
❑ supermarket   ❑ other (please specify)_____

Name_____

Street Address_____

City_____State_____Zip_____

GIVE ONE TO A FRIEND ...

Healthy Habits

are easy to come by—

IF YOU KNOW WHERE TO LOOK!

Get the latest information on:

- **better health • diet & weight loss**
- **the latest nutritional supplements**
- **herbal healing • homeopathy and more**

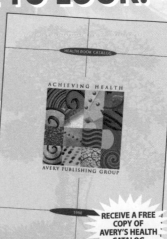

RECEIVE A FREE
COPY OF
AVERY'S HEALTH
CATALOG

COMPLETE AND RETURN THIS CARD RIGHT AWAY!

Where did you purchase this book?

❑ bookstore   ❑ health food store   ❑ pharmacy
❑ supermarket   ❑ other (please specify)_____

Name_____

Street Address_____

City_____State_____Zip_____

Avery Publishing Group
120 Old Broadway
Garden City Park, NY 11040

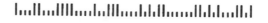

Avery Publishing Group
120 Old Broadway
Garden City Park, NY 11040